Occupational Therapy Practice in Psychiatry

LINDA FINLAY

CROOM HELM
London & Sydney

First published in 1988 by
Croom Helm Ltd
11 New Fetter Lane, London EC4P 4EE

Croom Helm Australia, 44–50 Waterloo Road,
North Ryde, 2113, New South Wales

Published in the USA by
Routledge, Chapman and Hall
29 West 35th Street, New York NY 10001

© 1988, Linda Finlay

Printed in Great Britain by St. Edmundsbury Press Ltd,
Bury St. Edmunds, Suffolk

ISBN 0 7099 49219

British Library Cataloguing in Publication Data

Finlay, Linda, 1957 –
    Occupational therapy practice in psychiatry.
    1. Man. Mental disorders. Occupational therapy
    I. Title II. Series
    616.89'1652
ISBN 0-7099-4921-9

Library of Congress Cataloging-in-Publication Data

Finlay, Linda, 1957–
    Occupational therapy practice in psychiatry/Linda Finlay.
        p.   cm. – (Therapy in practice)
    Bibliography: p.
    Includes index.
    ISBN 0 7099 4921 9
    1. Occupational therapy. I. Title. II. Series.
RC487.F54 1988
616.89'1652–dc19   88-20215 CIP

To Bob,
who advised and encouraged me
throughout the writing of this
book.

Contents

Use of terms

After much deliberation I have decided to refer to the patients/clients we treat primarily using the term 'patient'. This acknowledges that the majority of people we treat are still at present within the hospital system. Occasionally I have used the term 'client', but only when the context is clearly in the community. In recognition of the weight of the contribution of women within the profession of occupational therapy, I have referred, throughout this text, to the therapist by using the terms 'she' or 'her'.

Preface

Occupational therapy in psychiatry is often considered to be ill-defined in terms of its aims, imprecise in its methods and altogether too informal in its work practices. It can be seen as an area of our profession which is marked by a tendency to muddle through, rather than one which is clear about what it is doing and why it is doing it. This need not, and indeed should not, be the case. Admittedly, many issues in both psychiatry and occupational therapy are not clear-cut and there is certainly room for discussion and debate. However, if our work is to be effective it does need to be clearly specified and applied in a coherent fashion. We need to be reflective practitioners who work systematically through the stages of the occupational therapy process. We need to be clear about our aims of practice and our options for achieving them. We need to formulate and use clear frameworks to guide our practice. Only then can we begin to feel confident about, and able to articulate, what occupational therapy offers.

In this book I have tried to tackle these aspects by presenting occupational therapy as a problem-solving process that can be applied, clearly and systematically, as well as humanely. Chapter 1 takes an overview of our occupational therapy role, and in defining some of our specific functions it signals issues that are pursued in subsequent chapters. Chapter 2 lays down our theoretical foundations, illustrating the necessity for using some framework for practice. Chapters 3, 4, 6 and 7 logically progress through the occupational therapy process of assessment, planning, implementation and evaluation of treatment. Each of these chapters is designed to offer specific guidelines as to what the stage entails and how to carry it through. Chapter 5 extends the discussion on how to plan treatment and emphasises our special — even unique — role of using activity therapeutically. Chapter 8 concludes by examining a range of more general discussions and debates surrounding our present and future practice.

Throughout the book I have emphasised the practical application of occupational therapy. To this end, many case studies and practical examples are used; indeed the whole of Chapter 6 is devoted to a series of case studies. In addition, the majority of chapters contain some illustrative 'Theory into Practice' boxes which explicitly highlight these 'how-to-do' aspects of the subject under discussion.

I have also sought both to acknowledge and highlight those areas of our practice which are open to debate. It would be plainly wrong to attempt to offer some definitive statement of occupational therapy in psychiatry, given both the variety of practice that exists and our philosophy of unique, individual treatments. Thus while I often give my personal view, I have also tried to allow for differing standpoints. The discussion questions at the end of most chapters may prove fruitful in encouraging further thought, discussion and debate on these issues.

Having outlined what this book is intended to do I would like also to mention its limits. Somewhat reluctantly I have restricted its scope to the context of treating psychiatric patients and have not sought to cover the areas of mental and physical handicap. These are areas in their own right, which require full and separate treatment to do justice to the issues they raise. In mental handicap, for example, the issue is more about managing behaviour and teaching skills rather than giving treatment. In physical handicap, primacy is often given to motor function as separate from psychosocial aspects. Having said this, there are clear overlaps in all the areas — for example, our work in dealing with developmentally delayed children. Further, it remains true to say that the principles and processes discussed throughout, particularly those on structure of treatment and the need to evaluate, have a general relevance to all areas of occupational therapy.

In conclusion I would like to acknowledge a number of people who contributed to the making of this book. I wish to thank Paula Juffs, who has been one of the most significant influences on my thinking on occupational therapy over a number of years, for her helpful advice on reading my first draft. I am also grateful to Chris Mayers, who gave me the confidence to undertake this project, particularly in its earliest and most tentative stages. I also wish to express my thanks to Carol Walker, Anne Candelin, Tricia Yetton and Liz Holdich for their constructive advice and support. To all other staff and students (past and present) in the Occupational Therapy Department, The College of Ripon and York St John, who continue to stimulate and encourage my ideas — thanks. Finally, my gratitude needs to be given to both my general editor Jo Campling, and to Tim Hardwick, Senior Editor of Croom Helm, for their helpful comments on the completed draft. Needless to say, in the last analysis I alone remain responsible for any errors of content that may be found in the following pages.

Foreword

I was pleased to be asked to write a foreword to this book not only because the author is a valued colleague and friend but also because I believe this to be the most comprehensive, practical and realistic guide to good occupational therapy practice currently available for students and qualified therapists who work or wish to work with patients with psychosocial problems.

Too often in the past, those of us who work in psychiatry have been overwhelmed by the demands made on us and have abandoned some of our theoretical principles in order to try to adapt more quickly, but often less effectively, to the particular confused situations in which we have found ourselves. Sometimes the differing expectations of occupational therapists and the repeated questioning of our exact role have led to increased insecurity and a confusion in ourselves and others of how the occupational therapist's professional knowledge and skills should and could be appropriately used in practice.

In this book the author offers practical and realistic examples of how the essential theoretical frameworks and models which underpin the occupational therapy profession can be translated into effective and stimulating practice. Throughout, she engages the reader in a co-operative venture to improve contributions to care, encouraging us to explore current practice and to use the various discussion issues and rhetorical questions to reflect on how improvements may be made to that practice. The underlying theme is consideration of the occupational therapy process of assessment, planning, implementation and evaluation. The author presents each stage of that process in a comprehensible manner by showing how each has its theoretical justification, giving down-to-earth, step by step descriptions of how to follow through each stage, describing a number of examples of how this has been done in practice and finally by leaving us with discussion questions and opportunities for further reading. The emphasis throughout is on encouraging readers to undertake a systematic and specific analysis of our professional practice and on making us aware that all occupational therapy, however diverse its specialist areas may be, is contained under the same supportive philosophical and professional umbrella.

The book has three great strengths. Firstly, the author does make us reflect on our own practice and think about how we can justify our contributions to patient treatment programmes. She has given models which are so human and realistic that they cannot be ignored or brushed aside on the grounds that they are too idealistic. We are stimulated to improve by her example. Secondly, her comfortable and consistent reference to theoretical frameworks and models reminds us of our own need to become more familiar with the fundamental foundations of our professional knowledge and not to disregard them in our search for the innovative and the exciting. Thirdly, throughout the book we are aware of the essential humanitarianism of the author and of her deep respect for the individuality of each patient and the uniqueness of his or her needs. Comprehensive and academic though the essential theories and frameworks may be, they are presented as being valuable only in so far as they improve the occupational therapist's contribution to individual patients, clients or colleagues.

I believe we can all benefit professionally and practically from the empathetic and tireless work of this author.

Paula H. Juffs
York, January 1988

1

The Occupational Therapy Role

In this introductory chapter I want to perform three different tasks. First of all I will consider the role of occupational therapy in general, whatever the work context, in order to establish some basic principles. I will then apply these principles to the specific area of occupational therapy in psychiatry and, in the process, outline a simple model for practice which can be explored more fully in subsequent chapters. Finally I will try to convey something of the wide range and variety — of types of patients, problem areas, treatments — of practices encompassed by the phrase 'occupational therapy in psychiatry'.

OCCUPATIONAL THERAPY

In common with the majority of occupational therapists I have some difficulty in succinctly defining our profession. We can be involved in so many different areas, working with those patients impaired in physical, psychological or social aspects. We also carry out such a variety of tasks, from supplying a wheelchair to offering psychotherapy. Further, often the value of our work lies within aspects which are hard to quantify, such as the patient–therapist relationship or the satisfaction gained through activity.

In trying to construct such a definition here, we must bear in mind what it needs to cover. At the very least it should be able to specify the *aims* of occupational therapy. It also needs to indicate the *process* whereby the aims are achieved. Finally, and by no means least in importance, it should address the fundamental *beliefs* and values underlying those aims and practices.

1

Figure 1.1: The occupational therapy process

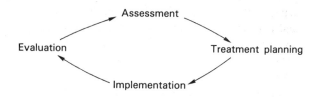

1. The main *aim* of occupational therapy is to assist individuals whose ability to cope with activities of daily living have been impaired by biological, psychological or social stresses. The primary occupational therapy concern is to help these individuals reach their highest *functioning* level — helping them acquire the knowledge, skills and attitudes necessary to perform their life tasks. Thus occupational therapists can be said to 'elevate the commonplace' (Yerxa, 1987), as we stress the performance of *skills* and tasks within the wider context of a person's work, social and domestic *roles*.

2. The occupational therapy *process* is primarily a problem-solving one (Hopkins and Tiffany, 1983). The first stage of the process is *assessment*, where we aim to identify an individual's problems of functioning. We then *plan treatment* by considering numerous options of what could be done to enhance the person's functioning. We consider the individual's skills, needs and lifestyle, and select the most promising problem-solving strategy that can be realistically applied, for the *implementation of treatment* stage. We then (and continuously) *evaluate* the treatment process, being alert to the need for further problem-solving if necessary (see figure 1.1).

   Two points need to be stressed about our kind of problem-solving. First, given the nature of occupational therapy work, the problem-solving process is not necessarily about 'solving' the problem in any simple or straightforward fashion. Rather, the best treatment solution may well be at the level of minimising the effect of the problem for our patients and maintaining their existing function. The second point I wish to emphasise concerns the *holistic* nature of the problem-solving process, i.e. treating people as complex wholes rather than homing in on an isolated part. Occupational therapists value this approach where all aspects of emotional, cognitive, social, physical, sensory and perceptual areas are acknowledged. As such, problem-solving addresses a very wide range of issues and necessarily encompasses a considerable diversity of practice in trying to resolve them.

3. Another way to understand occupational therapy is to recognise our fundamental *beliefs*:
   a) We believe that each individual has an inherent need for *purposeful activity*, i.e. work, play and rest occupations. In an occupational therapist's eyes a healthy person is one who is able to perform his or her daily occupations to a satisfying and effective level. This process can somehow be interrupted in the ill or handicapped person. We strive to ensure that our patients carry out these activities with a sense of competence that stems from them being able to perform the activities as efficiently as possible, feeling in control.
   b) This notion of the centrality of occupation underpins our view of the power and *therapeutic potential* of activity. We apply activities in the treatment process, valuing the activity's inherent properties, the experiencing of a 'doing process' and its end-products.
   c) Lastly, we value the uniqueness of each *individual*. Each person is seen to have his or her own skills and problems, needs and motives, and a wider social and cultural heritage. The implications this carries for occupational therapy is that each person requires his or her own individual treatment programme, which cannot be effectively used for another.

In summary, occupational therapy can be seen as a holistic, problem-solving process, where an individual's unique problems are treated through applying purposeful activity.

A SPECIFIC MODEL FOR PSYCHIATRY

How does the notion of improving function by problem-solving apply to the practice of occupational therapy in psychiatry?

In terms of trying to understand the types of problems we deal

3

with in psychiatry we can itemise the problems under the headings of emotional, cognitive, perceptual, social and physical. Alternatively, it may be helpful to look at three broad areas: feelings, behaviour and skills. (I use this latter formula most often in subsequent sections.) The 'feelings' problems commonly encountered in patients include: lack of confidence, fears, low motivation, unrealistic self-concept, unfulfilled needs, etc., as well as emotions such as anger, guilt and unhappiness. The 'behaviour' problems of patients (linked to feelings) include: withdrawal, apathy, passivity, aggression, hyperactivity and bizarre responses. The 'skills' problems suffered by patients encompass areas of task performance and cognitive skills (e.g. concentration, ability to problem-solve, physical ability), as well as as the more social aspects such as one-to-one communication and group interaction skills.

Of course these categories are artificial in that problems of feelings, behaviour and skills, experienced by an individual, usually occur together in a complex package. However, it is important to recognise that different therapists often focus on one type of area (e.g. the therapist concerned with teaching skills as opposed to the one who encourages self-expression). We will see later (in Chapter 2), how different theoretical commitments of occupational therapists may well produce a different problem focus.

It will be clear that when we look at problems we do not mean 'diagnosis' in the medical sense. Instead, we refer to problems of functioning that may occur in a person suffering an illness. For occupational therapists a person's diagnosis is primarily useful as an indication of possible problems and likely prognosis, and any precautions that may need to be taken. But we are less interested in specific symptomatology, and more interested in how the symptoms affect the person. Take, for example, two people with the diagnoses of depression and schizophrenia. From an occupational therapist's point of view they may well display similar functional problems: they may both be apathetic, passive and hypoactive in behaviour, have poor task performance skills and withdraw from social contact. These are the problems on which we would focus, resulting in the possibility of similar aims of treatment despite contrasting diagnoses.

Any list of such problems, however, is meaningless without reference to the individual's functioning in terms of wider life roles. Consider the two following cases, who might well benefit from the attentions of an occupational therapist. Our first case is

4

Figure 1.2: A model for occupational therapy practice in psychiatry

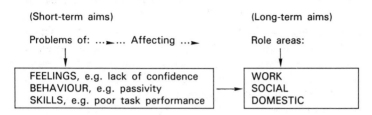

(Short-term aims)   (Long-term aims)

Problems of: ...►... Affecting ...►   Role areas:

| FEELINGS, e.g. lack of confidence
BEHAVIOUR, e.g. passivity
SKILLS, e.g. poor task performance | → | WORK
SOCIAL
DOMESTIC |

that of a student who, on commencing college, becomes anxious about social situations and withdraws. This sets up a vicious cycle which results in the student losing still more confidence in her ability to cope. Thus the interlinked feelings and behaviour problem begins to incapacitate her social life, and consequently her studies as well. Our second example is that of a shopkeeper who is unable to work due to the voices he hears. He cannot concentrate and makes mistakes, and his customers start avoiding the shop as they find his behaviour too odd. His problems of skills and behaviour functionally affect his work. These two studies show the need to understand people's problems in their own life context. Both individuals, for example, have problems of social skills; but they differ qualitatively and require different interventions. The student needs her confidence boosting and opportunities to experience successful interactions. The shopkeeper needs to be made aware of what he is doing, and given advice as to how to cope.

The occupational therapy problem-solving process in psychiatry can thus be seen as a focus on feelings, behaviour and skill which affect the role performance of individuals in work, social and domestic areas. We can illustrate this by means of a simple model (see figure 1.2), that also provides us with a framework within which we can identify an important distinction between short-term and long-term aims. In the short term we aim to enhance a person's immediate functioning (e.g. improve concentration). In the long term this is related to the person's life situation (e.g. rehearse work skills and resettle back to job).

In terms of the problem-solving strategies available we can use a multitude of *activities* ranging from work tasks (e.g. clerical or industrial), to social groups (e.g. dances, quizzes), to psychotherapy

5

experiences (e.g. projective art, psychodrama). We also use ourselves and our *relationship* with the patient as a key therapeutic tool, to encourage, support and activate our patients, and help them gain a more positive self-view. We also structure our treatment *environment* (people, equipment, surroundings) to facilitate the patient's growth or development. Thus our treatment can be seen as adapting and grading the activity, the therapist's role and the environment.

THE VARIETY OF ROLES IN PSYCHIATRY

So far (and throughout the rest of the book), I have avoided referring to different categories of patients and providing a treatment formula for them. This is appropriate given our emphasis on individual problem-solving. None the less, it would be unrealistic not to recognise that specific needs — and thus types of occupational therapy — are likely to be common to particular groups of patients. Indeed, only by attempting some schematisation can I hope to convey the wide range and variety of roles undertaken by occupational therapists in our work with psychiatric patients. For convenience we may group our patients into the following categories: acute admission; middle/long-stay (in hospital and being resettled); children and adolescents; elderly people; and other specialist areas.

Acute admission

Many occupational therapists work in wards/units of hospitals which could be termed acute admission. The patients' diagnoses vary considerably and include the more neurotic-type disorders and acute psychotic and affective disorders. Patients' ability to cope with everyday life is usually severely, though perhaps only temporarily, impaired, often by extreme feelings (e.g. of anxiety) or disturbed cognitive–perceptual processes, which affect their behaviour. The common factor is that the patients are usually discharged (or referred elsewhere) within six weeks.

This time-scale significantly affects our role, as therapy needs to be promptly applied. *Assessment* is usually an important aspect of the occupational therapist's (and team's) task. In a short space of time she needs to identify key problems/issues on admission, and then for discharge. On the treatment side, three types can commonly be encountered:

1. *Anxiety management* courses, where the patient can immediately learn practical coping skills of, e.g. relaxation;
2. *Group work* (e.g. drama or social skills training), where the patients share experiences and gain support and insight from each other and the activities;
3. *Craft/task* activities, for diversion, or promoting self-esteem and skills, or simply interest.

These more structured activities can also benefit those who are severely disturbed and find the 'containing' aspects useful. The key to applying these treatments for this group successfully, lies in our awareness of the short space of time available. We have to ensure that the patients get some rest (and perhaps space to be acutely ill), but also leave our care having benefited from a useful therapy package.

Middle/long-stay

The bulk of our work probably falls within this large group of what could be called middle- to long-stay patients. It encompasses some patients who have received treatment over a few months and those who have moved in and out of the hospital system over the years. In the main, such patients suffer from the continuing handicap of having a functional psychosis or an affective disorder. A range of other disorders may also be present, including some organic and personality disorders. The wide range of problems exhibited by this group often include a degree of institutionalisation where the patients tend to be more passive, dependent and apathetic, affecting all aspects of their behaviour. Their skills (in personal, domestic, work and social areas) often run the risk of deteriorating from lack of use. Associated problems include a much-lowered self-esteem and sense of identity, and occasionally 'sick-role' behaviour. These problems are further exacerbated by the appalling and hostile social environment (e.g. social stigma, unemployment, poverty, lack of social support) within which individuals in this group are commonly forced to live.

Our occupational therapy role with this group is likely to encompass virtually the entire range of our role options. Most commonly, however, we work on deficits of skills and behaviour (at least maintaining function) and focus on the following areas:

1. *Personal* — personal presentation and self-awareness activities, self-care or beauty therapy are mainstay activities;
2. *Social* — social skills training is widely used — otherwise, more diversional social contacts are encouraged;
3. *Domestic* — basic skills of home management are taught and practised;
4. *Work* — often sheltered work (e.g. industrial therapy or clerical work) practice and resettlement are used to offer a sense of role and structure for the day.

The theme of rehabilitation runs throughout all these sections, with particular attention being paid to finding optimum levels of stimulation to challenge and motivate (often the key problem), without undue pressure.

Middle/long-stay returning to community

This group is really a continuation of the previous category, but I have separated it out to highlight the recent community trend, which has had a fundamental effect on psychiatry as a whole. As a member of a multi-disciplinary team we may be involved in a community role carrying functions not previously mentioned. When the patient has been, or is being, discharged from hospital we may find ourselves involved in any or all of the following:

1. *One-to-one contact visiting the client at home* — here we have the general role of providing support on a continuing basis and it may include aspects ranging from encouraging the client to maintain their medication, to helping the individual structure their day. This latter function is particularly important when we recognise the often total upheaval of roles the person has had to make in moving to the community from hospital.
2. *Family contact* — some degree of family contact is likely, concurrent with visiting the client at home. Often success or failure of the person's integration back into the community depends on the family's ability and degree of motivation to give their relative support. Therefore, we may be involved in either general support or more specific therapy.
3. *Mobilising social support* — here, we often act as a referral

8

agent. This may be at the level of activating social services such as meals-on-wheels (when resources are available). More often it is a question of contacting relatives, day units, relevant voluntary groups (e.g. MIND), etc. to offer continuing social support. As part of this role we may also be involved in working in particular day units, which offer the service of maintaining the client's functioning and providing social contact.

Children and adolescents

Working with children/adolescents is a specialist area, though it appears to be a growing one of interest to many occupational therapists. Behaviour disorders are the most common diagnostic category found (e.g. including aggressive behaviour, encopresis, substance abuse). In recent times child abuse (especially sexual abuse) has become a major specialist area of particular sensitivity in public debate. In the case of adolescents there is often an overlap with concerns of adult psychiatry (e.g. diagnostically). However, whatever diagnosis is offered, what distinguishes this work area is the emphasis usually placed on the family as affecting or being affected by the child or adolescent. Similarly, attention is specifically focused on the schooling input, given the problems related to this area (for example non-attendance and developmental/educational delays).

Our occupational therapy input in this area of practice, varies between different units. Usually we work in four main ways:

1. Focus on feelings — non-directive playtherapy and projective puppetry are two ways of applying psychotherapy whilst using an activity medium. Children are encouraged to explore/play out feelings, helping them come to terms with their situation. The adolescents benefit in this way with group work (e.g. using drama and other projective activities).
2. Dealing with behaviour — we are often involved as part of the multi-disciplinary team (e.g. in a therapeutic community), in applying behavioural strategies (e.g. token economy or 'Time Out' procedures). In occupational therapy we may well have some groups of children/ adolescents carrying out an activity (e.g. cooking), as the focus for examining interpersonal behaviour.

9

3. Improving skills — we are concerned primarily with a child's developmental skills. Thus we may work on social, cognitive, perceptual or motor aspects, using play (e.g. sensory integration techniques encompass much of this).

4. Working with families — in some teams we may be involved with family work. This may include teaching parents play/parenting skills or participating in family therapy sessions.

Elderly people

A large area of our practice involves working with elderly people. In part we deal with this group on a regular basis within general psychiatry. There are also special units, largely dealing with individuals who have the diagnosis of dementia. With this group, however, general problems of ageing (physical, cognitive, social) are relevant throughout, as are the other psychiatric conditions of, for example, depression and anxiety. In many units we have the tail end of the long-stay population who have simply grown older in hospital. In each of these areas the problems and issues at stake combine to form a very different picture and fundamentally change our role. Thus in one unit our task may be solely assessment, and in another, long-term maintenance.

Our assessment role is a crucial one, where often we have to identify if a patient is 'safe' to return home. This typically involves cooking assessments, but also includes investigating general mobility, self-care, the availability of social supports, etc. We may also be called in to clarify a differential diagnosis, identifying the extent of confusion or memory loss, for example. Further, a *community input* is an increasing area of our work. This may be at the level of home visits to ensure safety. It also includes offering ongoing support at home, and referral to community centres (when resources are available). Contact with the relatives and voluntary agencies may be the crucial factor in maintaining a person's independence and dignity at home. In terms of activities, we may well be involved in *reality orientation* sessions (actively working on an individual's problems of memory loss, confusion and disorientation) or *reminiscence therapy* (encouraging social interaction). We also offer a range of general activities (sing-a-longs, bingo, keep-fit, crafts), designed to stimulate the senses, maintain function and provide enjoyment. In the last analysis when working with elderly individuals, we have a unique role to play, given our holistic training. Their physical problems cannot be separated from their emotional and social ones. We are well placed to offer a range of relevant therapy from perhaps advising on equipment, to bereavement counselling.

Other specialist units

Specialist units include areas such as substance abuse units, mother-and-baby units and forensic psychiatry. The diagnoses and problems encountered span a wide range as relevant to each unit, and are too numerous to mention here. Often, however, these day- or in-patient units deal with aspects of personality or behaviour problems (e.g. the history of violent behaviour found in many residents of secure units). The individuals concerned have usually found it difficult to cope within society's prescription of 'acceptable behaviour'.

In general terms we can identify the occupational therapy aims in such specialist units in three ways:

1. To operate as part of the multi-disciplinary team, where often in the more therapeutic community-type unit, the occupational therapy role is blurred with that of others. Group work can become a main role here.
2. To provide a range of relevant activities, for example cooking for enjoyment or to learn a skill, or gardening for its constructive and productive functions.
3. To teach relevant coping skills. A social skills training programme is often useful in, for example, teaching those with alcohol problems, 'how to say no to a drink in the pub', or teaching those inclined to violence, differences in being aggressive vs assertive.

DISCUSSION QUESTIONS

1. What are some of the key assumptions which underpin occupational therapy practice?
2. The values underpinning occupational therapy can be contrasted sharply with traditional medical values. Discuss.
3. Role blurring between the occupational therapist and other

11

team members creates only problems and confusion. Discuss.

4. In practice, can occupational therapy be said to be holistic?
5. Occupational therapy is unique in its use of purposeful activity. Discuss.
6. Given our limited resources, occupational therapists should concentrate their staffing on working with the middle/long-stay patients, as opposed to acute admission groups. Discuss.

2

Theoretical Frameworks

INTRODUCTION

This chapter is designed to persuade therapists who may be reluctant to explore 'theory' that some theoretical rationale is necessary to our profession and effective practice. I will do this by describing a range of theoretical frameworks commonly used in psychosocial occupational therapy, and highlight their practical application. These accounts will, of necessity, be in the form of brief summaries, but those of you whose interest is roused will also find that additional references are given to more academic and in-depth explorations.

On being asked 'How would you treat this patient?', you might well feel that the problem is not that great. There is obviously a 'right' analysis of the patient's problems and a 'right' treatment that flows from this. But things are not this straightforward. As this chapter will seek to persuade you, an important part of the answer to this apparently simple question will turn on a response in the form of: 'It all depends on whose theory I use.' Basically, a theory/model/frame of reference gives us our 'spectacles' through which we view our patients, their needs and problems, and the occupational therapy process. It helps us know what to look for and what to do, and gives us an understanding as to why we are doing it.

Before going into these questions, though, I would like to avoid some potential confusions surrounding definitions of terms by presenting the following simplified scheme which indicates how I am using the words:

Theoretical framework

Theory   = A system of assumptions and principles devised to analyse, predict or explain behaviour (or other phenomena).

Conceptual model   = A concrete representation of a concept that can account for certain data/relationships.

Frame of reference   = Our general orientation, a collection of ideas which provide a foundation for practice.

Philosophy of practice = Our fundamental beliefs, guiding percepts and values.

Why have a theory?

Theory, models and frames of reference are our 'mental filing cabinets' (Yerxa, 1987) which help organise our knowledge. More than this, they allow us to communicate our knowledge/understanding to others. Interestingly, we may well be using 'theory' unconsciously or by 'accident'. The usefulness of applying some theoretical base self-consciously, however, can be seen at a number of levels:

1. A guide to practice — when we are faced with the daunting task of treating another human being with all his or her complexities, our theoretical framework gives us a place to start, and a way of moving forward. Further, we need some theory base to encourage coherent and systematic treatment. Without it we risk 'synthesizing a plan for therapy that contains contradictory assumptions and modes of practice' (Briggs, Duncombe, Howe and Schwartzberg, 1979: 2). An example here is the use of reward star charts (behaviourism) with a child, whilst using non-directive playtherapy (humanism).
2. A guide to alternative practice — different theories often define the problems differently and suggest alternative treatment strategies.
3. A tool to encourage team co-operation — if we are ignorant of the theoretical biases within the team our opportunities to

blend treatment co-operatively, and to communicate effectively, are lessened. Any divisions between the team
members may arise because they are subscribing to different theoretical frameworks. Further, if we want to challenge
existing practice, we need to understand others' positions.

4. A way forward — a theoretical base provides both a
   rationale and method for documenting and researching our
   practice. This is vital, given increasing demands for
   accountability. 'A well-developed theoretical structure
   allows the therapist to meet questions from administrators,
   other professionals, families, clients and perhaps most
   importantly, questions that may arise from oneself as a
   therapist' (Fidler, 1985: 292).

What are our theoretical frameworks?

'Occupational therapists work under a myriad of theoretical
approaches or conceptual models' (Mailloux, Mack and Cooper,
1983: 284). On one hand we have a range of theories arising
from the biological and social sciences, which we have adopted
in our practice of occupational therapy. In psychosocial occupational therapy, for example, we have applied psychological
theories including: (a) psychoanalytical theory, (b) behaviourism,
(c) humanistic apporoaches and (d) developmental theories. On
the other hand, we have the currently powerful movement of
attempting to identify our own theoretical framework. The possible list here includes: (a) Reilly's occupational behaviour theory,
(b) Lloren's facilitating growth and development theory, (c)
Ayre's biodevelopmental theory, (d) Mosey's theory of adaptive
performance, and (e) more recently, Kielhofner's model of human
occupation. All these differing schools of thought have produced
a diverse range of practice. (For further discussion on the
desirability of many theories, see chapter 8.)

APPLIED PSYCHOLOGICAL THEORIES

In this section I will review the four main psychological
approaches commonly used in occupational therapy and discuss
their specific application. For convenience I will spell each out in
the form of a set of propositions.

The analytical approach

Basic concepts

The analytical approach arose primarily out of Freud's work in psychoanalysis with neurotic patients. Other theorists such as Erikson (critical life stages) and Jung (symbolism and collective unconscious) further enriched Freud's original work. Underpinning Freud's theory are five key assumptions. First, experiences in early childhood have a lifelong impact on personality. Second, humans have a large component of the irrational in their make-up and are beset by conflicts and anxieties and controlled by a dynamic unconscious. Third, development progresses through psychosexual stages (oral, anal, Oedipal, phallic, genital) during which points a person can become 'fixated'. Fourth, a person is seen as being determined by an interplay between his or her biology (instincts and id), psychology (emotions, ego, unconscious) and society (relationships and values). Fifth, and lastly, the therapist is required to make skilled and complex interpretations of individual case histories.

Application in occupational therapy

Gail and Jay Fidler were influential in the 1960s in bringing this psychodynamic approach into occupational therapy. Like other analytical theorists they stressed the role of the *unconscious* and *object relations* in influencing behaviour. Their theory and practice emphasised three other key points. They argued that *communication* is the essence of occupational therapy. They saw the inability to communicate effectively as the key psychiatric disability. Thus, in occupational therapy, the process and end-product of activities are designed to facilitate individuals to communicate thoughts/feelings which they cannot at a verbal level. They then stressed the importance of interpersonal *relationships* in therapy. In the treatment process both the patient–therapist relationship and the patient's interactions in a group are considered of central significance; for example for ego strengthening and reality testing. They further emphasised the *symbolic* and projective potential of activities which allow the expression and exploration of conflicts. Activities are seen as useful in dealing with self-concept; sexual identity; infantile, oral and anal needs; dependency; hostility and reality testing aspects. Their treatment process is generally aimed either at uncovering repression or support (Fidler and Fidler, 1963).

Theory into Practice
(Psychodynamic methods)

Assessment methods most usefully employed would be the observation of patients in a range of groups and activities, and projective activity. A typical analytical/psychodynamic assessment would include:

1. concept of self — e.g. self-esteem, body image;
2. concept of others — e.g. expectations, relationships;
3. ego organisation — e.g. defences, reality testing ability;
4. unconscious conflicts — e.g. needs, feelings;
5. communication — e.g. the nature of ability.

Some examples of *treatment* activities that could be used are:

self-portrait painting to develop a more accurate self concept;
cooking/eating to satisfy oral needs;
woodwork to express hostility safely;
structured sport to develop perceptions of self, movement and others;
discussion group to encourage a shared reality;
creative arts to facilitate sharing, awareness and communication.

The behavioural approach

Basic concepts

Behaviourism arose largely from the work of Pavlov (classical conditioning) and Skinner (operant conditioning). Their somewhat mechanistic focus on 'stimulus leading to response' and 'behaviour as a result of its consequences' has given way to a greater recognition by more recent theorists of the importance of social and cognitive aspects and other intervening variables. Common to all the theories, however, is their emphasis on three points. In the first place a stress is on observable behaviour. Behaviourists focus

17

primarily on overt behaviour rather than mental events. The therapist looks at what patients say and do, not what they feel. Any treatment should be targeted at breaking down old undesired patterns of behaviour (extinction) and developing new, desired patterns (through reinforcement). Secondly, behaviourists emphasise the process of learning. Primacy is given to the process of learning as a result of events in the environment. Positive reinforcement (pleasant rewards given) and negative reinforcement (removal of aversive stimuli) available in the environment, act to increasingly build a repertoire of behaviour. Finally, they are committed to a fully scientific approach. Fundamental to behaviourism is the active pursuit of a scientific methodology. Researchers attempt objectively to investigate behaviour in a laboratory, and use highly controlled procedures for modifying behaviour.

Application in occupational therapy

Occupational therapists have drawn widely on behavioural principles. We often apply them unconsciously/automatically, for example in our use of rewarding by praise. This has been more systematically explored by Mosey in our use of the *learning process* when applied to teaching patients basic skills (Mosey, 1986: 217–26). In its purest form behaviourism has been applied in many units — in which occupational therapists play a part — employing specific management programmes such as token economy.

Sieg (1974: 422) describes the process of designing a programme as involving five elements:

1. Identify the terminal behaviour desired (in precise and measurable terms);
2. Establish baseline data (what behaviour, when, how often);
3. Select *reinforcer* (to be suitable for the individual);
4. Select schedule of reinforcement;
5. Use techniques of *behaviour modification* (i.e. shaping, where successful approximations are rewarded; chaining, using step-by-step teaching; and modelling where successful imitations are rewarded).

Theory into Practice
(Behavioural methods)

Assessment methods rely heavily on structured observation.
Particular areas to observe would include*:

General behaviour
    appearance, e.g. posture;
    activity level, e.g. hyperactive;
    participation level, e.g. withdrawn;
    non-productive behaviour, e.g. rituals.
Interpersonal behaviour
    independence
    co-operation
    assertion
    sociability
    attention-getting behaviour.
Task performance behaviour
    co-ordination
    concentration
    following instructions
    activity neatness
    problem-solving ability
    organisation of task.

Treatment can be applied at two levels:
1. Behaviour therapy to modify maladaptive behaviour:
    a) token economy, e.g. to improve participation levels;
    b) backward chaining, e.g. to teach dressing skills;
    c) systematic desensitisation to decrease avoidance (of feared stimuli) behaviour.
2. Occupational therapy activities using applied principles:
    a) social skills training, e.g. to build a more effective social repertoire;
    b) anxiety-management sessions where relaxation, biofeedback and cognitive restructuring train new habits.

* Based on the Comprehensive Occupational Therapy Evaluation Scale — see Chapter 3.

The humanistic approach

Basic concepts

Humanism operates at many levels: it is an existential philosophy, an attitude towards therapy, and a particular approach to psychosocial treatment (Briggs *et al.*, 1979: 95). It covers a wide range of theories, including those of Carl Rogers (self-concept and unconditional positive regard) and Maslow (hierarchy of needs). Whilst the focus shifts between theorists, they would all concur about the importance of four basic elements. Firstly, they assign central importance to the self concept. The growth of the individual and the development of a healthy self concept are the key aims of therapy. The 'self' is explored (identity and image) and inner awareness expanded. Second, they stress the importance of human potential. An interest in human capacities such as love, creativity, individuality, autonomy and identity are seen as fundamental. Third, there is an emphasis on the fulfilling of needs. Individuals are seen to be motivated to fulfil needs for safety, esteem, love, productivity and actualisation. Finally, humanists place central weight on relationships. Relationships are seen as crucial in developing a person's self-esteem and image, as well as fulfilling needs. Thus they are a significant factor in therapy.

Application in occupational therapy

In occupational therapy the work of Yerxa is significant, as she explores what she sees as the essentially humanistic *values underpinning* occupational therapy; namely, our optimism, holism and approach to seeing the patient as active, autonomous and with a right to life satisfaction (1983: 149–60); 'by increasing the client's capacity to be independent we help him perceive himself as possessing worth. He is not a "thing" to be manipulated helplessly by others but is a human being who can exercise some control over his environment . . .' (Yerxa, 1967: 3).

Occupational therapy and humanism are also linked fundamentally, given the importance placed on our establishing a therapeutic relationship and in our use of activities. At one level our prescription of activity to maximise potential, excite creativity, and improve self-esteem, applies to much of our work. At another more specific level the range of *creative therapies* (art, drama, dance, writing) we employ, arising in part out of Gestalt therapists and Moreno (psychodrama), provides the classic example of humanistic theory in action.

Theory into Practice
(Humanistic methods)

As fitting with the philosophy, any *assessment* relies heavily on the patients' own subjective accounts, eliciting their perception of reality. Thus, much use is made of counselling interviews and self-rating questionnaires. Typical questions that might be asked include:

Self concept — how do patients view themselves, their strengths and weaknesses? What discrepancies exist between the real and ideal self?
Needs — what needs and feelings are particularly strong at the moment? What are the patient's goals for the present and future?
Situation — how effectively are the patients' basic needs being met in their work and leisure pursuits? What is unique about a patient, given his or her age, gender and sociocultural background?

Appropriate *treatment* media include:

dramatherapy to play, express, share oneself;
printing to achieve and create;
beauty therapy to improve self-image and esteem;
non-directive counselling to become more aware and grow;
free play to explore self and the world with freedom;
dressmaking design to express individuality.

The developmental approach

Basic concepts

A multitude of theories embrace a developmental approach. Freud, or Erikson or Piaget could all be said to utilise such an approach. Thus there is no one theory that speaks definitively on the subject. Some theories, like Piaget's cognitive development, focus on one area. Others, like Mosey's (adaptive skills), are multi-dimensional and attempt to encompass all aspects of development. The basic principles shared by all can be summarised as five points. First, 'development' is the orderly progression of an individual through a series of complex, interacting stages. Second, an individual grows and learns in a sequential way — each gain provides the base for the next. Third, there are qualitatively different problems and opportunities that emerge at each stage, and need to be mastered. Fourth, under stress or illness, individuals can regress to previous stages. Finally, treatment involves identifying the particular functioning level and providing experiences to facilitate step-by-step learning and adaptation (applied learning).

Application in occupational therapy

Occupational therapists are especially concerned with all aspects of development, and it is a concept to which we continually refer. We apply our knowledge of 'normal' expectations to facilitate development in those impaired. This is achieved by applying a teaching process of:

1. providing success experience that confirms stage learning;
2. encouraging safe exploration, then practice to move forward;
3. providing opportunities for challenge.

Anne Cronin Mosey's theory of adaptive skills presents us with a comprehensive example of both the *sequence* of development and how to intervene therapeutically. She outlines six areas of functioning or 'adaptive skills' (note that this is a revision from her previous work proposing seven skills), which are further divided into subskills. These subskills give us the specific 'ladder rungs' or goals to use in the teaching/learning process. Mosey's six adaptive skills are:

1. Sensory integration skill — the ability to co-ordinate vestibular, proprioceptive and tactile information for functional use.
2. Cognitive skill — the ability to organise sensory information for problem-solving.
3. Dyadic interaction skill — the ability to engage in a variety of one-to-one relationships.
4. Group interaction skill — the ability to participate in a

variety of groups.

5. Self-identity skill — the ability to perceive self as a relatively autonomous, acceptable person who has continuity over time.

6. Sexual identity skill — the ability to perceive one's sexual nature as good, and participate in a mutually enjoyable, long-term sexual relationship (Mosey, 1986: 416–42).

When treating a patient it is not possible to work on all these areas, though a focus on one area usually prompts growth in another. Some units (e.g. the Maudsley and Bethlem Hospitals, London, in the late 1970s), have organised their occupational therapy programme highlighting one adaptive skill (see summary example figure 2.1). In using the example of group interaction skill, the process is one of: 1) identifying a newly referred patient's skill level; 2) slotting them in the appropriate level group (one that is both safe and offers challenges); and 3) facilitating 'higher' behaviours.

Figure 2.1: Summary of group interaction subskills

18 months–2 years   Parallel group level = able to work alongside others in a group.

2–4 years   Project group level = minimally shares, competes and co-operates with therapist prompting.

5–7 years   Egocentric–co-operative group level = co-operative and competitive, experiments with group roles.

9–12 years   Co-operative group level = meets needs of other members and expresses both positive and negative feelings.

15–18 years   Mature group level = flexibility in taking on various roles within a heterogeneous group.

23

Theory into Practice
(Developmental methods — group interaction)

Assessment would take the form of structured observation using a developmental checklist of skills of group interaction. Individuals would be placed in a series of non-threatening groups (e.g. craft group, cooking, volleyball game) to be observed. If they showed some awareness of, and could work alongside, others, though they seemed unable to share their tools, the patient would be placed in a project-level group. If, during the volleyball game, the patient showed the ability to take turns and be competitive, then a higher-level group would be required.

Treatment — assuming the individual was placed into a project-level group, the main aim would be for the therapist to encourage co-operation and sharing between members. The group of six to eight patients would ideally meet daily for one hour to perform a variety of task and social activities. The therapist would carefully grade the environment by encouraging the group to work in pairs sharing tools, and then as a whole, around one table. When members showed they had learned the relevant skills they would be promoted to another group.

AN ILLUSTRATIVE CASE STUDY

By now you may well feel puzzled, or even frustrated, by this account of rival theories suggesting different approaches. 'What does it all mean in practice?', you may well be asking. So let us proceed to answer this by way of an illustrative case history.*

Peter, aged 30, had been in hospital for one year with a severe schizophrenic illness. He presents as extremely withdrawn, regressed and confused. His behaviour is bizarre, as he often

---

* The account of the case study and subsequent treatment are fictional and have been produced for learning purposes only.

spends time curled on the floor or rocking stiffly in a chair mumbling to himself. At these times he can become physically aggressive if attempts are made to move him. Peter seems to lack awareness of himself, as evidenced by his behaviour and unkempt appearance. Currently, on the ward, the nurses have to do much for his basic care, and during his withdrawn phases they even have to feed him. During his admission, sporadic attempts have been made to get him involved in occupational therapy, often without success, and prompting verbal abuse, though on occasions he will wander into the occupational therapy department and sit passively in a corner. The team have decided to make a concerted attempt to engage Peter in an active rehabilitation programme, and it has been suggested that the occupational therapist become the 'key worker'.

How would four therapists of different thoeretical persuasions tell their own story about how to treat this same patient? As you will see, whilst they each use the medium of pottery, they mobilise very different approaches and aims, and these ultimately are shaped by, and depend on, their theoretical commitments.

The analytical approach

The occupational therapist's assessment highlighted Peter's (a) aggression — possibly a lot of underlying anger, (b) regression and dependence — indicating his current needs and (c) limited communication — signalling his need for another channel. Her priority in treatment was to develop a nurturing relationship, where Peter could feel safe to engage in activity and begin to express himself.

1. The first stage of treatment was a daily visit to the ward to make contact with Peter — she gently spoke to him without asking for a reply;
2. One day she brought with her a piece of clay, and whilst talking, she made a small figure, and asked if Peter would like it — he nodded;
3. Subsequently, the therapist met with him regularly, talking and playing with the clay, either on the ward or in the department when he showed up;
4. He soon became involved with the claywork, gradually using bigger pieces.

25

Earlier, the occupational therapist had chosen claywork as it offered a means to make contact and for Peter to regress (with the messiness of the material). Now it was being used projectively, as a way of expressing feelings and channelling aggression (e.g. wedging the clay) — being destructive in a controlled way. Later, treatment would be geared to maintaining the therapeutic relationship and exploring other areas.

The behavioural approach

After assessing Peter, the therapist highlighted three problem areas: (a) self-care, (b) passive behaviour and (c) lack of social interaction. It was decided that the nurses should focus on self-care, whilst the occupational therapist would attempt to 'activate' Peter and engage him in some constructive task behaviour. Discussions revealed that a cup of coffee would be an excellent reinforcer, as Peter loved this drink but was rarely able to have it on the ward.

1. Initially, Peter received a cup of coffee for coming down to the occupational therapy department and staying for half an hour, which proved a highly successful invitation. At these times the therapist stayed with him for increasing periods whilst playing with a piece of clay. When Peter began to show an interest by also playing with the clay, she praised him.
2. On the next day, when this occurred, she suggested he have his cup of coffee earlier than usual, when he made something. Subsequently he only received coffee when he had used the clay for a period.
3. Increasingly, Peter spent more time with the pottery on his volition. After a few weeks, and some occasional instruction, he produced some attractive pots, and as he earned a good reputation he began to actively seek instruction and increase his skill.
4. This led to the next phase of treatment, which was to encourage active and appropriate social behaviour.

The humanistic approach

The occupational therapist's assessment highlighted a two-fold concern for Peter; namely, a lack of self-identity, as associated with his illness and as a result of being in an institution, and lack of any creative self-expression. On the positive side she felt his occasional unsolicited attendance at the department indicated his possible interest, and an attempt to make contact. On reviewing his social background she discovered Peter's past hobby of pottery and clay sculpture.

1. On the next few occasions Peter arrived in the department, the occupational therapist spent a few minutes sitting with him without making demands. She said his name, and made comments about the environment. She also indicated her impression that he might be interested in joining some time in the future.
2. One morning, whilst maintaining her consistent approach of gently talking to him, the occupational therapist fiddled with a piece of clay. Increasingly, Peter joined in manipulating the clay. No attempt was made to ask him to 'make something', they just worked side by side.
3. Whilst he remained quiet verbally, in action he tentatively played and interacted with the therapist, through the clay.
4. As their relationship developed, Peter began to talk, and be more independently involved with the pottery. The next stage would be to involve him in other creative activities with some wider group/social input.

The developmental approach

The occupational therapist's assessment findings indicated problems in all areas of development. Peter was found to be functioning at a severely regressed level in the social (one-to-one and group), cognitive and self-identity areas. His sensory-motor functioning was also problematic, given his stiff curled posture, limited body movements and apparent lack of body awareness. This latter area seemed an appropriate point of focus.

1. Peter was actively encouraged to come down to the occupational therapy department and work on a one-to-one basis

27

with the therapist, in a quiet space, free from distractions. She initially engaged him by asking his 'help' in making a large coil pot.

2. With general physical prompting and verbal encouragement, Peter was helped to make some large coils and cover them with slip.

3. After several coil pots his skill, enjoyment and involvement grew daily, and he graduated to other projects which used his initiative and larger movements more (e.g. stirring the glaze bin and wedging the clay. Throughout, the therapist was supportive and maintained a directive approach of giving instructions and reminding Peter to focus on the task.

4. When a consistent routine of doing pottery was established, the treatment plan was to progress on to additional physical activities (for gross movement) using the gym and sports equipment.

DISCUSSION AND MORE THEORIES

During the course of this chapter we have explored why we have to employ a theoretical framework, and some of the theories that are available for our use. The practical applications of four psychological approaches — analytical, behavioural, humanistic and developmental — were illustrated by a case study. Here the hypothetical example of the same patient, and four different treatments, allowed the approaches to be compared and contrasted. Thus I hope to have shown the profound and subtle influence of theory on how we 'understand' patients' problems, and how we apply treatment.

All this leads us to ask the obvious question: which is the best theory? Many of our problems would be solved if I could give you a simple or straightforward answer to this. Unfortunately life is not that simple! All the theories have their own strengths and weaknesses. The answer to this question will depend in part on the criteria you bring to bear. The analytical approach is based on a rich, comprehensive theory, and offers much scope for exploring inner feelings and the dynamics underlying mental illness. Its weakness remains its abstract, unproven assumptions, and the practical constraints of applying it in general practice. The behavioural approach, in contrast, produces tangible results

Table 2.1: Summary of four theoretical frameworks

Theory	Key concepts	Application in occupational therapy	Case study example: treatment
Analytical	Dynamic unconscious, psychosexual stages, needs/drives/conflicts, relationships/communication	Expression/exploration of inner feelings, symbolic/projective potential of activity	Aggression, regression and dependence worked through using the relationship and projective quality of clay
Behavioural	Learning, observable behaviour, reinforcement from environment, scientific methodology	Behaviour therapy, social skills training, relaxation techniques, teaching skills/behaviour	Passive behaviour treated with coffee as a reinforcer for task-orientated behaviour
Humanistic	Growth of the individual, self concept, human potential, feelings/needs/relationships	Values underpinning occupational therapy, creative therapies, activity used as positive experience	Self-identity and creative expression encouraged through relationship and creative/play quality of clay
Developmental	Defined sequential stages through which an individual grows — many different theories	Step-by-step teaching of adaptive skills, focus usually on one area	Sensory integration aspects worked on using tactile stimulation and gross movements of claywork

in behaviour change, and relies on proven, systematic methods and scientific research. Its weakness is its potentially rigid focus on small pieces of behaviour to the detriment of the whole person. By way of contrast again, the humanistic approach takes this idea very much on board, recognising human nature, its needs and potential. The assumptions of humanism are mirrored in our occupational therapy values, but is its applied treatment a little too vague and unrealistic? The developmental approach is logical, informative and well-structured. But given its wide base, if you focus on one area, what happens to the rest of the problem areas? In any case, whose developmental theory should we use?

In choosing between theories we not only need to look at their contrasts, but also to recognise the similarities regarding both their views on the nature of humans and the meaning of activity. Note, for example, how both the analytical and developmental approaches take a slightly biological view of humans and define growth through stages. Observe also how psychodynamic and humanistic occupational therapists use activities as self-expression, whilst the behaviourists and developmental therapists stress learning skills.

In practically applying theory we have a choice of committing ourselves to one particular theoretical approach, or working eclectically (drawing on a range of approaches). Often this choice is guided by our own leanings, the theoretical bias of our unit or the methods in vogue at the time. In practice we also choose the framework to suit our particular patient's needs. If, for example, the patient's priority problem concerns 'feelings', then a psychodynamic or humanistic approach would be suitably applied. If, on the other hand, the patient lacks certain behaviours and skills, the behavioural and developmental approaches can be brought into operation.

Whatever 'choice' we make should be an informed one, where we understand the strengths, weaknesses, similarities and differences among the theoretical approaches. An awareness of other approaches acts as a healthy challenge and critique of our own practice. Then, with knowledge, we can carry out appropriate, coherently applied treatment.

One point that needs to be made now, is that we have by no means examined all the theoretical approaches available. Instead I have discussed those approaches which have an established foothold in the United Kingdom, and which can be keenly contrasted. Whilst the four main theories discussed all have a good grounding in accepted psychological theory, I am not advocating they are the best, or the only, way forward. It is interesting to note in this context that, in the United States particularly, there have been attempts to develop theories which are not so much borrowed from other disciplines, but arise out of occupational therapy itself — relating specifically to our concerns. So to conclude this chapter I will briefly highlight four such currently influential approaches.

Llorens — facilitating growth and development

Llorens has been influential in asserting that occupational therapists should work from a developmental perspective. She sees occupational therapy as a process of facilitating growth, and mastery of self and environment, through recognising the abilities and needs of a child (1970: 93–101). As with Mosey's theory, the principles have then been applied to adult psychiatric patients. Her theory can be summarised as shown in table 2.2.

Table 2.2: Principles of Llorens' theory

First-level intervention — acquisition of 'supportive skills and behaviours'	Second-level intervention — acquisition of adaptive functional ability in 'occupational performance'
Sensory (perception and integration)	
Cognitive integration	Work
Motor co-ordination	Education
Interpersonal — social skills	Play
The ability to relate to human and non-human objects	Self-care
The ability to respond to and effectively interact with the environment as required by culture	Leisure

Reilly — occupational behaviour

Mary Reilly, of the California group, fought to return occupational therapy to its original notions of purposeful activity and intrinsic motivation to engage in activity. Basically, her occupational

31

behaviour model is concerned with the following four themes. In the first place a person's *life roles* (e.g. player, student, worker, retiree) are seen as stretching over a developmental continuum. Any therapy should pivot on looking at expectations of the role and associated task demands. Secondly, she emphasises the *balance* of life experiences (temporal adaptation); namely, work, play and self-maintenance. Third, *play* is significant in developing the knowledge and skills necessary for the life skills. This occurs initially by exploring, then developing competence, and striving to achieve. Finally, Reilly takes a 'systems' view in which individuals are strongly influenced by their environment (receiving stimulus and gaining feedback).

Ayres — bio-development theory

The research of Jean Ayres (1963: 221–5) into the development of sensory-motor function has led to the significant technique of *sensory integration*. Whilst remaining a specialist area it has gained a worldwide influence with its application to:

1. Learning-disordered children and mentally handicapped people;
2. People diagnosed as having schizophrenia, given their perceptual and postural problems (King's extensive work);
3. Those with traumatic neurological lesions (Bobath's work).

The basic principles underlying sensory integration are three-fold. First, early vestibular, tactile and proprioceptive experiences are important in personality development. Second, perceptual processes are crucial for the individual to adapt to the human and non-human environment. Lastly, carefully chosen *motor and sensory activities* can be effective therapy for those with deficits in their integration. Activities can be recreational or task-orientated, involving gross movements, vestibular stimulation, sensory input and awareness of space and form. King also notes that the patient's attention should focus on the activity object and not on the motor process, and that the activity should be pleasurable (1974: 529–36).

3

Assessment

Assessment is the first stage of the occupational therapy process, and consists of gathering information in an effort to understand the patient and his or her situation. In terms of a problem-solving process it is the vital stage of trying to understand the problem — not only what the problem is, but how it affects the person or others involved.

This chapter aims to explore different aspects of the occupational therapy assessment process. Firstly, by answering the questions of why? what? when?, assessment is put into a context. Secondly, methods of assessment are described and their use considered. Lastly I will discuss a range of practical, ethical and more philosophical questions about assessment, recognising the wider implications of it in practice.

WHY? WHAT? WHEN?

Why do we assess?

Careful, accurate assessment is vital if effective treatment is to be applied. After all, how can we know what to treat, and to what level, if we have not specifically identified the area of need? Further, how can we treat people as individuals if we have not discovered what is special about them?

As a problem-solver the occupational therapist needs to be clear about the problem and its parameters. Consider the therapist who is referred a patient who 'lacks concentration'. In order to plan treatment, she needs to find out:

1. What exactly is meant by this? What happens (e.g. lapses into non-productive behaviour)? When does this occur (e.g. during tasks)? How does this affect the patient's functioning (e.g. unable to return to the task)? Here the problem is specifically defined.
2. How long can the patient concentrate now in general functioning (e.g. five minutes)? This is the baseline to measure any improvement.
3. What situations increase/decrease concentration? This is important for both the patient, when developing strategies to cope better with the problem, and the occupational therapist to plan a graded treatment.
4. What level of concentration ability does the patient require for daily living? For example, a university student about to take exams, and a long-stay patient likely to remain in hospital, require qualitatively different levels. This information is needed to establish the aim of treatment.

If these questions are not answered the resulting treatment stands in danger of being stereotyped (i.e. not recognising the individual's needs), 'waffley' (i.e. lacking specific goals), and possibly completely ineffective (e.g. may end up working on the wrong problem!). In all, assessment is important in order to: (a) understand the problem/s, (b) recognise the person's individual needs, (c) identify the baseline for treatment and (d) evaluate future progress.

What do we assess?

As the first stage of the occupational therapy process, assessment involves the gathering of information, from any relevant source, about the patient and his or her circumstances. Importantly, each member of the treatment team is similarly involved in an assessment process, though they may have a slightly different focus according to their role and concerns (e.g. the doctor might home in on symptoms more). Whilst occupational therapy assessment is designed to clarify functional problems concerning a person's life roles, it also fundamentally seeks to highlight any strengths and positive areas from which to build (see figure 3.1). Thus we consider the person's problem areas and strengths in the context of their particular lifestyle and situation.

Figure 3.1: Bases of occupational therapy assessment

We assess:

The problem/s Regarding: person's skills, behaviour, feelings — functioning in general	+	The person Including: interests, needs, strengths/assets (e.g. skills, supportive family)	+	The situations a) Person's life roles (at home, work, play) b) Expected environment they are going back to, including support systems c) Social/ cultural aspects that may be relevant e.g. religion

When do we assess?

Assessment occurs at all points during treatment — initially, subsequently and continuously (see figure 3.2). At the initial stages the occupational therapist (and whole treatment team) will be involved in collecting data — observing, interviewing, testing the patient (and possibly the family). The information that is collected will then be analysed (preferably with the patient) to consider the priority problems and central issues to be dealt with during treatment. Further specific assessments may then occur at set times according to need; for example every fortnight, or prior to discharge home. At the continuous level, however, assessment is ongoing throughout treatment. This is often an automatic, intuitive process where the therapist is alert to the patient's responses and any new cues.

METHODS OF ASSESSMENT

There are many different types of assessment available for our use — some standardised and formally recognised, some simply prac- tised locally. Basically we have five main methods, other than general observation, of eliciting information about a patient, his or her problems, skills and situation: (a) interview, (b) specific observation, (c) standardised tests, (d) self-rating methods,

37

Figure 3.2: The assessment process

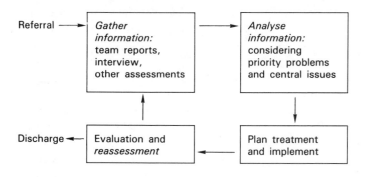

(e) projective activities. These will be described considering their aims, design and the type of information they can elicit.

Interviews

Interviews are the use of conversation to gain insight into a person's world. They are most widely used as our initial assessment tool, and often they remain the only more formal procedure the occupational therapist will apply.

Aims

The main aim of the interview is to gain information from the patient, considering both what he or she says, as well as how he or she says it. At a verbal level we are concerned to tap relevant factual information (e.g. situation, interests), feelings/attitudes and the patient's own view of problems. We can also obtain information regarding verbal skills and intellectual capacities. At a non-verbal level the patient's appearance and behaviour may communicate much about mood, mental state and attitudes. What specific information we seek to gain depends not only on the patient's specific problems, but also on the type of interview, therapist aims, patient's ability and his or her motivation. Different interviews do different jobs. Thus the interview that takes place as the first contact between therapist and patient is primarily a relationship-building exercise, with the occupational therapist sharing as much information about her role as the patient shares about his or her situation. Subsequent treatment-planning interviews will have a more specific focus regarding the patient's attitudes, interests, and view of problems he or she is prepared to work on.

Design

Any interview must be planned carefully, considering its specific aims and structure, as well as other factors such as the environment and the patient's previous experiences. Prior to the interview the therapist should be clear about what she hopes to achieve and why, whilst also being flexible to the needs of the situation. Is the interview primarily relationship-building? If so, the emphasis should perhaps be on a more informal basis (cups of tea and tours around the occupational therapy department are occasionally helpful here!). Is the interview more a fact-finding mission? Here the therapist can usefully go into the situation armed with a few already formulated, pertinent questions. This pre-empts vague interviews, and can help in those moments when we 'go blank' and do not know what to ask next.

The structure of the interview process itself is, of course, determined by its aims. In general, however, there are two important guidelines:

1. Be an active listener (more easily said than done), where effort is put into listening instead of formulating your next question.
2. Ask open-ended questions, such as 'How are you settling in?', as opposed to 'Do you like this ward?', or 'What does your typical day look like?', as opposed to 'Do you have a job?'. This way of asking questions allows a person more opportunities to expand his or her comments, and open out, rather than responding with a 'yes' or 'no' answer. Further, it implicitly respects our patients' capacity to take responsibility to share what is important to them. A possible exception to this, however, is when an acutely ill person seems to need the structure of a direct question.

As a general rule the environment should be fairly relaxed and safe, in order to encourage the patient to feel comfortable and open up. Often a quiet room off the main ward, or similar area, which the patient is familiar with, is a good start. 'Safety' and trust is also promoted by giving enough time, and being free from interruptions.

Theory into Practice
(Ten useful interview questions)

1. How are you settling in the unit?
2. Can you tell me a bit about yourself/your home/work?
3. What does your typical day look like?
4. How does your depression/anxiety/hearing voices affect your everyday life?
5. What difficulties have you been having lately?
6. What do you consider to be your strong point/talents?
7. What do you want to change about yourself?
8. What do you see yourself doing six months from now?
9. Have you ever had any contact with occupational therapy before?
10. What hobbies or interests do you have?

Other factors to consider include the patient's skills and past experiences. One rather thoughtless institutional practice, for example, arises when a patient is a given number of interviews by several professionals, all asking similar questions. Consider the not-uncommon occurrence of the newly admitted acutely anxious patient, who in the first week may be seen for an initial interview by several doctors and nurses, as well as a range of therapists with their attached students. We need to strike a balance between checking information from previous reports, showing an interest and gaining useful information. It is important for the occupational therapist to decide the particular focus of her questions in view of her particular role (e.g. questions about current problems in functioning would be more relevant than questions about the quality of delusions, on which the medical staff would focus).

Specific observation

Observation is of course the method of assessment we are using all the time. We continuously, often without thinking, monitor (and then respond to) how our patients are presenting, behaving and performing. We try to note how they are reacting to others, their activity and the environment.

The therapists who are particularly skilled at observing, learn to focus on specific and relevant cues. Thus, general observations like 'John is looking better today', are transformed into 'John's posture is more upright today, making him look more confident'. It is this level of specific observation which we need to encourage in ourselves, for two main reasons. Primarily, if we are more specific about a patient's areas of skills or behaviour we then have a more specific baseline for treatment. A second, not unimportant, factor concerns our professional presentation and our communication with other staff. Thus our occasionally vague, verbal reports can have far-reaching negative consequences.

To help us observe more effectively it is often helpful to utilise some of the infinite number of observation checklists available (see Appendices 1–3). Many of our *activities of daily living* checklists, for example, can be a useful prompt to highlight points, such as in the following:

Making a cup of tea   *Comment*
    aware of use of equipment
    organises task in sequence
    aware of safety factors
    fills kettle appropriately
    turns on gas/electricity switches
    puts tea in pot/cup appropriately
    pours boiled water in appropriately
    uses sugar/milk appropriately . . .

Further, we can take any developmental chart and translate it into behavioural forms, giving us a clear focus. The following example, detailing the *cognitive function* at a two- to three-year-old level, show this:

                                    Date achieved   *Comment*
    draws vertical lines
    copies circle
    matches three colours
    points to big/little in imitation
    places objects in, on and
    under on request . . .

41

An excellent scale used primarily for initial assessment observation is the Comprehensive Occupational Therapy Evaluation (COTE) scale (see table 3.1). (This has been used widely in the United States and is largely standardised (Hemphill, 1982: 211–26). (It is also currently applied in the United Kingdom, under a variety of disguises.) In addition to the basic scale there are official definitions attached, detailing the problems at a specific level to maximise reliability, as the following example shows.

> 1. A. Appearance — the following six factors are involved: clean skin, clean hair, hair combed, clean clothes, clothes ironed and clothes suitable for the occasion.
>
> *Rating*: 0 = no problems in any area; 1 = problems in one area; 2 = problems in two areas; 3 = problems in three or four areas; 4 = problems in five or six areas.

The form has been designed for flexible usage, being an observation checklist, a record of performance over time and an acutal report which goes into the medical notes (providing other team members understand the references).

The value of a specific observation form such as this is that it can be applied to many situations and tasks and, providing it follows a fairly standard practice, helps an objective account (though it cannot be called standardised unless accepted procedures are followed). A patient's actual functioning can be observed rather than inferred, which is the key issue at stake. For example, it could be used to assess a patient who is making a cake within a baking group. Here the patient's general and interpersonal behaviour can be observed as it occurs. The task behaviour can then be linked to relevant sections, e.g. following directions — does the patient follow demonstrated instructions (easiest), verbal instructions, or does he or she read the recipe? How much assistance or repetition does he or she need?

Table 3.1: COTE scale

Name . . . .

Date . . . .

	0	1	2	3	4
1. *General behaviour*					
A. Appearance					
B. Non-productive behaviour					
C. Activity level (hypoactive or hyperactive)					
D. Expression					
E. Responsibility					
F. Punctuality					
G. Reality orientation					
Subtotal					
2. *Interpersonal behaviour*					
A. Independence					
B. Co-operation					
C. Self-assertion (compliant or dominant)					
D. Sociability					
E. Attention-getting behaviour					
F. Negative response from others					
Subtotal					
3. *Task behaviour*					
A. Engagement					
B. Concentration					
C. Co-ordination					
D. Follow directions					
E. Activity neatness or attention to detail					
F. Problem-solving					
G. Complexity and organisation of task					
H. Initial learning					
I. Interest in activity					
J. Interest in accomplishment					
K. Decision-making					
L. Frustration tolerance					
Subtotal					

Scale: 0 = normal, 1 = minimal, 2 = mild, 3 = moderate, 4 = severe.

Comments

Therapist's signature

Standardised tests

A standardised test is a formal procedure which has been carefully researched and practised, increasing its objective and scientific status. Three main elements must be addressed when standardising a test:

1. The test norm must be defined — i.e. the accepted standard given a particular population needs establishing;
2. A consistent, clear administrative procedure and scoring system needs to be developed and used by specifically trained assessors;
3. The instrument's validity and reliability must be established (i.e. does the test measure what it is supposed to in a consistent way, across assessors and time?), with many trials and possibly adjustments

Most of the assessments we use in occupational therapy are not standardised. This does not negate their value, but should alert us to the importance of approaching any results with caution, and indicate that we need to ask further questions such as 'how did you arrive at this result?' Importantly, with some time and research applied, many of our tests currently in use can achieve the 'standardised' label. The pool of standardised tests available, however, is increasing yearly, with our emerging awareness of the need for specific, valid, reliable assessment. Some of the more widely known assessments in the United Kingdom are the 'Clifton', 'Rivermead' and 'REHAB'. Two standardised assessments well used in the United States are the 'Bay Area Functional Performance Evaluation' and the 'Interest Checklist'.

CAPE

The Clifton Assessment Procedures for the Elderly were developed by psychologists A. Pattie and C. Gilleard (1979), for their own use, plus 'all those professionally concerned with the care and management of the elderly'. The procedures are simple tests consisting of two scales designed to assess cognitive and behavioural competence:

1. The cognitive assessment scale measures knowledge/orientation (by quiz-type questions), mental ability (by counting, reading etc.) and psychomotor skill (by tracing a spiral maze).

2. The behaviour rating scale considers physical disability, apathy, communication and social disturbance. Comparison of the results with available norms allows the therapist to assess the degree of dependence present, indicating the levels of care and support needed.

This package can be obtained from NFER-Nelson Publishing Co. Ltd, Darville House, 2 Oxford Road East, Windsor, Berkshire, SL4 1DF. This firm will supply standardised tests to named individuals qualified to use them, and also offers demonstration workshops if needed.

The Rivermead

The Rivermead Perceptual Assessment Battery (Whiting, *et al.* 1984) is one of the main standardised perceptual tests available for occupational therapists in the United Kingdom. It consists of a battery of 16 timed tests (taking approximately one hour to administer). Tasks range from matching simple pictures to copying a complex three-dimensional model. The test is designed to measure deficits in visual perception, and as such has greatest application in assessing patients with neurological disorders. The attached manual includes information on interpretation of scores, and illustrative therapy case studies. This battery can also be obtained from NFER-Nelson (see above).

REHAB

The Rehabilitation Evaluation Hall and Baker (Baker, 1986) is a broad assessment package encompassing aspects of disturbed behaviour, work skills and daily living skills (social, self-care and community skills). Basically it is designed to gain a profile of patients through observing them in rehabilitation settings. The scale is growing in use, particularly as it can be applied by a range of professionals. Hall and Baker have studied large numbers of long-stay psychiatric patients, and offer a comparison between the individual's score and that of the 'peer' group. They found this information useful when allocating patients to different settings (Baker, 1986: 12–40). The scale and scoring guides can be obtained from Vine Publishing Co., 2A Eden Place, Aberdeen, AB2 4YP.

Bay Area Functional Performance Evaluation

This package is an assessment battery involving interview, structured and projective tasks, and observation rating scales. The two subtests assess task performance and social interaction. These provide information about affective, interpersonal, cognitive and perceptual-motor areas, in terms of daily living tasks. It has been well researched and is considered reliable and valid (see Hemphill, 1982: 255–307). The package and instructional videotape is available from Consulting Psychologists Press Inc., 577 College Avenue, Palo Alto, California, 94306, USA.

Interest Checklist

The Interest Checklist (Matsutsuyu, 1969) aims to assess a person's leisure interest and experiences. Eighty activities are listed, against which the patient indicates casual, strong or no interest. This self-rating inventory should be supplemented by discussion. This classic checklist is widely used, and has been modified to suit different people and treatments.

As with all standardised tests, in order to avoid their common misuse/abuse three points need stressing.

1. It is important that the assessors are properly trained to administer and score the test according to standard methods, maximising the test's reliability and validity. As more tests are published, and are generally available, we need to question whether they are being used as originally intended. There are courses available that train therapists in the use of specified standardised tests (enabling a person to become eligible to administer a restricted number of tests). For further information contact the College of Occupational Therapists, 20 Rede Place, London W2 4TU.
2. Testing is not just a matter of following procedure; it also requires interpretation of results. Here the occupational therapist requires a good understanding about the rationale behind the test and the comparisons with any available norms. Without this the test remains an observational tool only.
3. Be aware of the limitations and weaknesses of each particular test. Tests are usually designed for specific populations, types of problems and/or situations, and are

only applicable to such areas. Some tests are weak in certain areas, such as being vague with their instructions. The result will be an invalid and unreliable test if not administered precisely. A further point to recognise on some tests is the performance tensions which can arise and unduly affect the result.

Self-rating methods

These assessments involve the patient in formally completing a rating scale or questionnaire (or similar). The self-rating method is used in a variety of ways and can measure the patients' own perceptions of themselves, their attitudes, feelings or their interests (See Appendix 4). The main aims of this assessment are to gain information 'straight from the horse's mouth', so to speak, and to involve the patient actively in his or her own treatment. The range of diffferent self-rating tools available carry with them a range of differing aims and structures. Four brief examples will be given, with their different implications for use.

Hobby interest checklist

Please tick which of the following activities interest you most:

pottery
dressmaking
woodwork
watching television
playreading
gardening
sport
cooking
typing . . .

Notes. This type of form is often best used in the early stages of treatment, where a lot of information can be recorded, stored and possibly used towards planning treatment. They are forms which can easily be filled out by the patient to cover 'factual' information quickly. Care must be taken, though, not to dehumanise the process, reducing our patients' view of themselves to a few ticks. Thus some discussion, or other ways of using the form, subsequently will increase its value.

47

Work assessment form (weekly record)

Apply rating criteria of 0 = no serious problems, 1 = some problems, 2 = definite problems needing further help:

Skill area	*Patient rating*	*Staff rating*	*Comments*
. . . accuracy			
speed			
neatness			
organisation			
coping with			
pressure . . .			

Notes. This is an example of an ongoing evaluation form where the patient is actively monitoring his or her own performance in co-operation with the therapist. The aim of this method is to increase the patient's awareness and involvement, therefore improving motivation. If large discrepancies arise, they are interesting in themselves, or may highlight the need for further observations. This type of form, is perhaps best used on a regular basis (e.g. during weekly interviews) with the same therapist providing consistent standards to allow for measuring any improvements.

Social anxiety rating scale

Select the choice of difficulty which most closely fits how you feel about the following social situations: 0 = no difficulty, 1 = slight difficulty, 2 = moderate difficulty, 3 = great difficulty, 4 = avoid area.

Situation	*Date*	*Date*
. . . going to parties		
going into restaurants		
meeting strangers		
initiating a conversation		
maintaining a conversation . . .		

Notes. This is an example of a behavioural rating scale which could be used prior to social skills training (see also Appendix 4). Its value lies in how it specifically pinpoints the person's problem area. As the material is potentially emotive, care needs to be taken on presenting this to a patient. It is perhaps best used within a counselling-type interview, where answers can be expanded on and discussed. If the questionnaire can be filled out honestly (given a safe therapeutic relationship), then it can act as a valuable baseline to which the patient can subsequently refer, confirming progress (hopefully!).

Self-concept questionnaire

Please circle the appropriate answer. I would like to learn:

. . . that I am a person of worth and value	yes	no
to be less self-destructive	yes	no
to feel better about my appearance	yes	no
to feel I am competent . . .	yes	no

Notes. A range of self-rating tools like the one above have been designed in an attempt to grapple with patients' views of themselves and their emotional responses. They are particularly valuable for promoting insight, and can be useful when comparing the person's own view with that of others. Given their nature they are potentially threatening, and are certainly not easy to complete. At the very least patients may have difficulty with the jargon, or in confining abstract concepts to yes/no responses. Moreover, patients may not be ready to apply such concepts to themselves (e.g. may lack the insight). Given these potential pitfalls, much care must be taken both in choosing patients who would find this technique useful, and in presenting it to them in a caring, sensitive way. Often the tests are best used within ongoing counselling sessions or as part of a personal 'diary' in which an individual monitors his or her own feelings more privately.

Thus a range of self-rating questionnaires/forms exist, and they are adaptable in how they can be used by both therapist and patient. In summary, they can act as: (a) a motivator, where the patient can be active in his or her own treatment; (b) a casual checklist, to touch on verbally or in writing; (c) a vehicle for further discussion/counselling; (d) written evidence, to refer back on as treatment progresses; (e) a tool, to promote insight and awareness; (f) an opportunity to explore the patient's own view of the world compared to that of others.

Projective activities

Projective tests arise primarily within the analytical framework and are designed to tap deeper feelings and unconscious material.

Table 3.2: Summary evaluation of types of assessments

Type	Assesses	Value/strengths	Limitations/weaknesses	Implications for use
Interview	Most areas: e.g. general information regarding: life situation, self-perception attitudes, interests, behaviour, mood, etc.	Patients can communicate what they feel is important Relationship-building Facts and subjective aspects	Responses often depend on skill of therapist regarding: asking right questions, being sensitive/listening etc. Patient can lie Patient may not be skilled verbally or is withdrawn/ uncommunicative	Be clear about aims of interview and questions to ask Important to develop skills of active listening
Specific observation	Primarily skills/ behaviour, e.g. task performance, kitchen assessment, self-care, group interaction	Judgements made on basis of what seen/ performance, not on inferences or patient's assurances; therefore fairly objective More practical/activity-based so fitting our role	Validity/reliability still not assured as it relies on therapist observation skills and accurate interpretation. Limited contexts for observation Less able to identify subjective experience	Consider standardising form/task Recognise limitations of observation and continue developing skill Draw on observations over time/place/people
Self-rating	Primarily: Feelings Attitudes Interests Self-concept, etc.	Taps more abstract, subjective experience Patient allowed to communicate what he or she feels is important. Respects patient's capacity/responsibility for treatment	Patient can lie Can be impersonal Certain forms may threaten, irritate or be too abstract	Use as vehicle for growth/ development Use selectively and sensitively Consider using forms flexibly, e.g. patient fills it out privately and chooses what to discuss

Standardised tests	Many areas, often: behaviour, work or cognitive/perceptual/ motor skills	Scientific validity/ reliability heightened. More 'official', so often more respected by both patients and colleagues Baseline for research	Can be impersonal and anxiety-provoking Value lost if incorrectly applied Assessor should have special training	Strict adherence to standard practise important Times before and after testing important for relationship-building and feedback
Projective activity	Feelings, attitudes, self-concept, relationships	Taps more abstract, subjective experience Relationship building Can be therapeutic in itself (e.g. increasing awareness/insight)	Responses depends on therapists' skills with medium Can be emotionally painful/threatening and at times contraindicated. Patients may 'produce' what they feel is expected Temptation for therapist to overly interpret or infer	Careful selection of patients and activities Avoid interpretations, always ask/confirm what patient wants to say Feelings expressed need to be dealt with, not just assessed. Allow time

The tests rely heavily on the interpretive and analytical skills of the therapist. Since their conception they have been adapted and remoulded to suit the needs of various therapies. In the United States some projective tests have been standardised, such as the Azima Battery and the Shoemeyen Battery (Hemphill, 1982: 57–86). Whilst occupational therapists in the United Kingdom do not generally use formal projective tests, we have taken some of their principles and devised a range of psychodynamic activities that can be used for assessment purposes. These activities, though not standardised, provide us with a wealth of information about our patients, their feelings, needs and hopes and, as such, need to be included within this section.

Projective art

One example here is painting on two halves of a paper: 'an aspect of myself I dislike, and an aspect of myself I like'. Not surprisingly, people with a low self-esteem find the latter task, of acknowledging something they like about themselves, difficult. As such, this is also a useful exercise in therapy, and occasionally the therapist may have to insist that both sides of the paper are completed. If done in a group, this kind of exercise can also greatly aid self-exploration, particularly when parallels are drawn between the group members.

Creative writing

One activity that could be used here is writing 'a friend's description of me'. This particular technique is an attempt to elicit a self-view which is more difficult to write in the first person. The exploration of self-concepts, as seen by others versus self, is a further elaboration that can be fruitful.

Play therapy

Commonly, a doll's house can be used to explore family dynamics. A point of interesting debate that arises in this (and other) methods is whether or not everything the child plays out has a meaning. Whilst psychodynamic theory would say 'yes', pointing to symbolic meanings, I feel we need not be so dogmatic. Instead, we can say that sometimes a child's play can be extremely revealing, with the play being either a reflection of family life or a form of wish-fulfilment.

Theory into Practice
(Case examples — types of assessment)

1. *Ann*, a housewife, aged 56, is depressed, labile and says she is a failure. Assessment methods:
   a) counselling interview;
   b) observation of presentation and skills during cookery group;
   c) self-concept questionnaire.

2. *Thomas*, aged 76, has a possible diagnosis of dementia. Assessment methods:
   a) interview including questions requiring memory;
   b) CAPE;
   c) family interview.

3. *Jamie*, a boy of six, with an apparently deprived childhood, has been referred because of destructive behaviour. Assessment methods:
   a) observation of play in one-to-one and group situations;
   b) projective art, 'draw your family';
   c) discussion with teachers.

SOME ISSUES FOR DISCUSSION

In this chapter I have mainly advocated the use of fairly *formal*, specific assessment, over the widely practised *informal* methods. The key reasons I support these are two-fold: the effect of our own prejudices, values and idiosyncrasies can be reduced by standard routines; and any specific assessment focus promotes a clearer understanding of central issues both for the patient and other treatment team members. What is your view?

The therapists who primarily support the often-intuitive unstructured ways of assessing patients would find a number of arguments against using formal approaches, such as: 'Specific assessments are too artificial, cold, mechanical, and put the patient under stress. The important thing is to get on and treat the patient, we don't have the time to assess constantly — and have we the right to judge? . . .' In this section some of these debates will be aired, acknowledging their wisdoms, whilst also challenging their assumptions.

Science obscuring art?

Is occupational therapy in danger of losing its essentially humanistic values in bowing towards the pressure of science? For example, what justification is there to put a patient under stress in the name of objective data? The classic example of this is a task assessment, where a patient is allowed to fail as the occupational therapist wants to observe how he or she manages without reassurance or assistance.

I would certainly agree that we need to remember 'the person' behind the 'subject to be assessed'. We must not destroy the 'art' of maintaining a therapeutic relationship in the name of 'science'. But perhaps we are being grossly unfair to the scientists, who also need to maintain a rapport with their subjects. On a task assessment, for example, where the patient may be put under pressure, the therapist would of course take care to be supportive both before and after, if not during (as she may need to eliminate variables such as giving assistance). The patient needs to know what he or she and the therapist are doing, and why. Further, the therapist should be flexible enough to jettison the task if it is creating undue problems — another form of assessment may be more appropriate.

In debate I would also raise another point: that the prime purpose of assessment needs to be borne in mind — the gathering of information which will ultimately help the patient with more effective treatment. In this case the more secure we are about the accuracy of that information, the better. 'Science' in this sense is more about being systematic and trying to ensure as much accuracy as possible. Thus the basic answer to the science versus art dilemma probably involves finding a balance.

Making judgements

Do we have the right to make judgements about patients — particularly on the basis of one or two formal assessments? My view is that we have to make judgements, and they cannot be avoided. The judgements we make, however, should be contained within the limits of 'professional requirements, and not our personal moral standards, religious beliefs or political views. Whilst we are entitled to have and advocate these, we should not subject our patients to them.

How we make judgements is the issue of immediate practical importance. The following points are some ideas towards making judgements more effective and constructive.

1. Try to be as objective as possible, to limit the possibility of being blinded by stereotyped perceptions. Here we especially need to guard against being swayed by labels, diagnosis, etc., which could act as self-fulfilling prophesies (e.g. when working with institutionalised patients, reducing aims to the lowest common denominator). The debate of whether or not we read the patient's case notes prior to the initial meeting is particularly pertinent here. It is probably an individual choice according to how swayed we might be. I personally prefer to form my own initial impression of the patient prior to reading the notes. A brief report from the other team members (e.g. asking if there are any precautions I need to be aware of) first, however, is a useful compromise. I would also want to know the type of questions the patient has already been required to answer in the other team members' interviews.

2. Acknowledge any gaps or limitations in your judgements to avoid possible misinterpretation. A constructive example here is: 'Mary is safe using our department cooker. Further assessment is required to confirm her safety at home'.

3. Devote more energy to collecting data rather than making inferences. For example, consider the potential trap we may fall into when we see a patient cry, and find we make interpretations that he or she is inadequate or being manipulative (see figure 3.3).

4. Constantly monitor judgements/assessments to confirm, deny or adjust to changing circumstances. Here the team can well use each other by sharing impressions on the basis of a patient's 24-hour day. Certainly we need to be wary of making firm judgements of limited evidence. Using solely one or two tests is potentially problematic, unless we limit the scope of what information we are trying to gain.

5. Acknowledge any assumptions of what is 'normal' or 'desired behaviour', which lie behind many of our judgements. This is

Figure 3.3: False interpretation of data

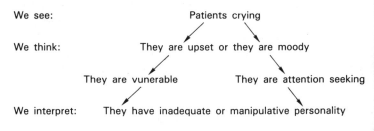

We see: Patients crying

We think: They are upset or they are moody

        They are vunerable   They are attention seeking

We interpret: They have inadequate or manipulative personality

particularly important over time as views and fashions change. Also we each have our own cultural standards which may be highly relevant (e.g. in notions of moral behaviour).

Best use of scarce resources?

A common complaint given against assessment is 'we do not have the time or staffing available to do extensive one-to-one assessments'. Certainly, this reality is a large stumbling block. At the risk of answering glibly, however, it would seem to be about choice of priorities. Do we prefer to treat more patients and do less assessment, and run the risk of supplying vague treatment? Or do we prefer to assess each patient in order to ensure some degree of individual treatment planning? Furthermore, at all points of treatment we have to make choices about which patient has priority over another, and how. It may well be impractical to consider lengthy in-depth assessments for every patient. Therefore, we have to:

1. Select only the patients who seem to be at an apppropriate stage for the kind of occupational therapy available. The other team members' reports are useful here.
2. Select the most useful assessment method to use, given the patient's skills and problem areas, and the therapist's abilities.
3. Select the area on which occupational therapy should focus specifically. Here is where the team need to work together (e.g. the nurse focusing on personal-care skills whilst the occupational therapist considers the home environment and the social worker considers the family supports).

Another question I have heard posed in this context concerns the possible dangers of spending too many resources on assessment whilst never getting down to treatment. I would agree that there is a danger of occupational therapists 'over-assessing' — spotting the problems without considering problem-solving. Often this is a result of feeling assessment is a clear, valuable role; therefore, therapists develop their skills in this area, and treatment time is diminished. It is worth considering this further, however. Isn't assessment part of treatment? A key part of interviewing, for example, can be the use of counselling techniques. Also the deeper one-to-one contact of intensive assessment may have more remedial benefit than longer 'treatment' consisting of being in a large, more casual group. In the end, though, the only justification for purely playing an assessment role is when specific recommendations for treatment/follow-up elsewhere are made.

The patient's experience

Often we are faced with a dilemma about how to present assessment to our patients. If they are aware of being observed/assessed, won't that alter their performance? For example, it may make them more nervous or inclined to put on an act. Can we not unobtrusively observe? Should patients be aware of what we are trying to do? Further, should the results be shared and discussed openly?

Clearly there is no definitive answer to these questions, as it depends on the individual patient, the type of assessment, the chosen team approach, and possibly our own inclination. In general, though, we have two guidelines — legal and moral. At the legal level we are under increasing pressure to begin to open up to our 'consumers' (e.g. Data Protection Act). The New Mental Health Act also emphasises this, when saying some information should be accessible to the patient. Without the legal argument, however, we perhaps need to return to our basic philosophy of recognising the notion of handing responsibility over to our patients. If they are to take an active part in their treatment they need to be aware of the aims of treatment, which of course emerge out of the assessment. Thus a degree of openness would seem essential from the start. Maintaining a 'professional silence', or finding devious ways of uncovering problems, works against encouraging mutual trust.

If a patient is overly threatened or anxious on being observed/ assessed, we need to consider the situation further. A number of factors may be involved. Firstly, the patient may feel that he or she is being judged negatively. Here the problem would seem to lie more within how the therapist is presenting assessment in the first place. Alternatively, the patient may feel a certain amount of natural 'performance tension' on being given set tasks. We, of course, must take this into account and consider the patient in several contexts over time. Lastly, we may be inadvertently appearing too distant or threatening, e.g. by our non-verbal behaviour. The writing of notes during assessments is an example of this, and whilst it is perfectly acceptable practice, it has a negative side if human contact is broken.

In my view, where possible our patients should have some control over what information is gleaned from any assessment, and how. They need to be encouraged to alert us about what is important to them, and what they wish us to know. As always, our best way of considering the patient's experience is to confront how we would like to be treated.

DISCUSSION QUESTIONS

1. To what extent is assessment a part of treatment?
2. What criteria should we use to decide which assessment methods to use?
3. What are the strengths and limitations of each method of assessment?
4. To what extent should occupational therapists consider the scientific method in assessment?
5. What is meant by reliability and validity, and why are these important?
6. Various psychological theories are implicit within each assessment method. Discuss.

4

Planning Treatment

Planning treatment is a process involving the organisation of information in such a way that the patient's problems are identified and treatment principles, goals and activities are specified. It is a logical procedure where aims of treatment follow on from problems identified. It can also be an exercise in lateral thinking where, in the design of treatment, we consider a wide range of possible ways of enhancing a patient's functioning, before settling on the most practical option. In essence this involves three stages — spelt out below — and it is an excellent maxim to write these out explicitly in your patient's notes, as a clear guide to the treatment you are undertaking. The three stages are:

1. *Organising the information* — information obtained from assessments is organised to highlight problems and priority areas.
2. *Establishing aims and goals* — the overall aim, plus short- and long-term aspects.
3. *Designing the programme* — grading the activity, therapist role and environment to meet aims.

The process needs to be seen in the context of the overall plans of the treatment team and, as such, involves some team liaison and negotiation. Failure to do this can lead, for example, to an unnecessary duplication of therapy between nurses and occupational therapists over a patient with 'poor self-care'. Unless properly organised in terms of 'extra reinforcement', two different programmes are a waste of resources and could possibly be confusing for the patient. It is most important that such team negotiation and treatment planning be done in conjunction with the patient. At a basic level this may simply mean the patient expressing a preference between two activities; at its fullest extent the patient may be encouraged to take full responsibility for his or her own treatment planning. Let us now examine each of these three stages of treatment planning in greater detail.

ORGANISING THE INFORMATION

There are four key elements here: processing the information, identifying the problem, identifying positive aspects and selecting the priority problem.

Process the information

In the initial stages of planning treatment a considerable amount of information arising from the occupational therapy assessment findings, and other team members' reports, etc., needs to be processed. In addition, factors regarding the clinical condition and practicalities of treatment will also need to be considered. In summary, the range of information that needs to be taken into account includes those shown in Table 4.1. Some of this information is, of course, more relevant than other data for the occupational therapist. In-depth knowledge about the diagnosis, for example, while interesting, is less important than a recognition of how the disorder is affecting the patient's functioning. Again, past medical and psychiatric history is of less concern to occupational therapists, than is recognising the 'expected environment' of the patient, which will influence his or her future roles/needs.

Table 4.1: Range of information

Occupational therapy findings	Team members' reports	Practical aspects
General functioning of patient	Clinical condition and prognosis	Limits on treatment such as time and resources available
Social, domestic and work circumstances	Past and present treatment	Theoretical frameworks employed
Expected environment	Past medical, psychiatric and social history	Treatment media available

Identify the problems

After sifting through the available information the occupational therapist needs to identify the problems. Given our primary role as problem-solvers, the task of highlighting problems accurately, is a crucial one. It is useful to draw up a problem list, and the more specific its content, the better. The occupational therapist is especially concerned to highlight problems in functioning, e.g. those listed in table 4.2.

Table 4.2: Problems in functioning

Problem	Description	Effect on function
1. Poor task performance	Unable to carry out simple task independently — concentration and sequencing particularly affected.	Dependent in dressing; unable to cook safely
2. Passive	Does not initiate action or conversation unless prompted	Dependent on others for basic self-care; isolated

Identity positive aspects

Any successful treatment must build in an acknowledgement of the patient's strengths, interests and motivations. The patient's strengths need to be stressed as often we use his or her skill in one area to help the problem area (e.g. a creative bent being harnessed to learn a craft to improve task skills). At the very least we need to remind the patient (and ourselves) of his or her positive points to help balance our emphasis on problems. The patient's interests should be taken into account as part of appreciating his or her social and cultural background and needs. The process of incorporating strengths and interests usually goes some way to aiding the patient's motivation to engage in treatment or activity (a crucial variable if treatment is to be effective).

Select priority problem(s)

Realisitically, we are rarely able to treat all the problems identified in assessment. Firstly, occupational therapy cannot be a

61

panacea for all ills. Secondly, if we tried for a comprehensive coverage of problems, our treatment would stand in danger of being far too wide ranging. Consider for example, the chronically institutionalised patient, who has received minimal therapy in recent years. The problem list is likely to be long (possibly encompassing: stooped posture, unkempt appearance, hypoactive and passive behaviour, poor reality orientation, poor social skills, low motivation, poor concentration, difficulties in carrying out tasks etc.). In the initial stages it would be impossible to work on all of these problems. It is far better to select a particular area for focus. This may then have additional positive benefits, rather like a dominoes effect (e.g. figure 4.1).

Figure 4.1: Positive benefits of selecting key problems

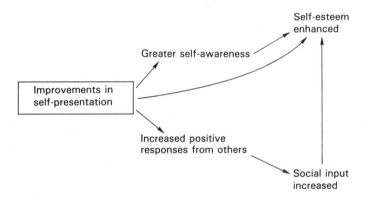

The skill of the therapist, then, lies in the selection of a few key problems to work on initially. This can be done on the basis of several criteria:

1. Select the most basic or underlying problem, e.g. poor social skills may be at the root of the difficulties of a person who is having problems in both relationships and finding/keeping a job.
2. The patient could be invited to arrange the problem list in a hierarchy. If the patient is working on what he or she perceives to be important, then the motivation is likely to be higher.

3. The family or staff could select an initial problem which they see as over-shadowing all other aspects, e.g. commonly behaviour which is overtly bizarre or out of control needs to be managed before any fine-tuning is attempted.
4. The problem which has an easy solution could be worked on first, as part of confidence-building in the therapist–patient relationship, e.g. teaching relaxation techniques for coping with anxiety or supplying a communication aid, immediately.
5. Lastly, an important criterion is the influence of whichever theoretical framework is being used, e.g. therapists in the humanistic tradition are more likely to select problems of feelings as being fundamental, whereas behaviourists would direct their attention to behaviour.

Theory into Practice
(Example of negotiating the problem)

Therapist. During this interview, Jean, you've mentioned a number of problems ranging from what you're feeling inside to the strains of work and home.

Jean. Yes, everywhere I turn there seems to be another problem.

Therapist. (nods, acknowledging Jean's comment) I think we'd find it difficult to work on all those problems at once. Is it possible to narrow them down a bit to see if we can come up with one or two areas to work on first?

Jean. I guess so, (unsure).

Therapist. Okay, let's see . . . which problem causes you the most stress? or which problem do you want to get rid of the most? or which problem has the most/least effect on your life?

Jean. Oh I don't know . . . . I can't cope with the children and their screaming . . . . The biggest problems are at home, I'm so tense . . .

Therapist. Yes. One of the things we find in therapy is that sometimes, if you get one problem area sorted out, the other problems sort themselves out too. For example, if you were feeling less tense, do you think you might cope with your children's screaming better?

Table 4.3: Aims of treatment

Levels of aims	Examples
1. To improve the problem area or develop/increase skill	Develop conversation skills
2. To maintain skill or prevent deterioration	Maintain existing social skills
3. To minimise the problem or help adjust to difficulties	Encourage non-verbal methods of communication to compensate

ESTABLISHING AIMS AND GOALS

We now come to the second main stage involved in planning treatment, namely, establishing aims and goals. Once the problem(s) to be solved (or minimised) have been identified, the aims of treatment should follow logically from them.

Treatment aims often deal with the problems at different levels as table 4.3 demonstrates.

A logical structure to use when devising aims/goals could follow the pattern of: establish the overall aim, identify short- and long-term aims, and then set specific goals.

Establish overall aim

This aim, established by the team (and constrained by available resources), provides the basic direction of treatment, e.g.:

1. to discharge home resuming an independent life; or
2. to undertake graded rehabilitation aiming for discharge to a sheltered environment; or
3. to improve the quality of life whilst the patient remains in hospital.

With this aim being clearly stated, further aims can be realistically constructed.

Table 4.4: Short- and long-term aims

Short-term aims	Related long-term aims
1. Improve task performance skills of concentration, sequencing, following instructions, attention to detail, etc.	Ensure safe level of cooking skills prior to discharge home.
2. Learn relaxation techniques. Become more aware of the importance of non-verbal behaviour. Demonstrate increased confidence in conversation ability	Practise skills of being interviewed prior to going to actual situation.

Identify short- and long-term aims

Whilst acknowledging the grey area between 'short-term' and 'long-term', a simple formula can be applied to emphasise their differences. Basically, short-term aims refer to improving immediate function/skill or working on the components which make up the wider life skills (e.g. general/interpersonal behaviour or task skills). Long-term aims consider these problem areas in terms of a person's life roles (e.g. work, social and domestic aspects (See table 4.4)). (Note that the two examples in table 4.4 also demonstrate the difference between therapy-centred and patient-centred aims — both are used in practice.)

Set specific goals*

Having established an aim, you will now require a more step-by-step account of what it entails and how it is to be achieved. Goals are precise statements of intended results, and serve as realistic, measurable targets for both patient and therapist. The effective goal includes what is to be achieved, and how, plus the criteria for measuring its achievement. For example, the aim 'to improve the ability to concentrate' can be transformed more precisely into the goal of 'at the end of a month of regular practice, Mr Brown will be able to concentrate a minimum of 20 minutes on a basic familiar task.' (Subgoals might include: at the end of the first

---

* 'Objectives' often used as a synonym.

Theory into Practice
(Setting goals)

A systematic desensitisation programme designed for a person suffering from agoraphobia is a classic illustration of sequential goals, e.g.:

1. Walk to the front gate with therapist, then alone without anxiety.
2. Walk ten steps outside gate, with therapist, then alone, without anxiety.
3. Walk to the corner shop, with therapist, then alone, without anxiety, etc. . . .

---

week . . . five minutes; second week . . . ten minutes, etc.)

The following points should be remembered when establishing aims and goals. First, aims and goals should always be written down. Unspecific, mental goals are insufficient. It is too tempting to devise them retrospectively. Once written they can act as something tangible to work towards, and can also be more easily communicated to relevant team members. In the second place goals should, if possible, be negotiated with the patient. At the very least their agreement is needed to ensure their co-operation, and hopefully motivation. Further, the process of negotiation may in itself be therapeutic, e.g. trying to establish realistic goals with a person who has an unrealistic self-concept. Thirdly, goals must be achievable. Whilst the overall aim of treatment may require a large leap in the patient's functioning (e.g. from being 'ill' to being 'well'), it is essential that the patient feels he or she can manage the immediate mini-steps. Herein lies the difficulty, however, as there is a fine balance between underestimating the patient's capacity (which results in boredom), and overestimating (which may result in failure and loss of confidence). Because of this, room for failure might need to be built in as 'understandable' or 'acceptable'. Fourth, goals should be flexible in adjusting to the patient's needs and performance. They therefore need to be regularly re-evaluated with the patient. Lastly, it should be noted (and the discerning reader will have done so) that on certain occasions it is inappropriate to set goals. This is particularly the case when working in the more psychodynamic traditions. The humanistic approach for example, of letting the client lead (e.g. in non-directive counselling), leaves little room for the therapist to structure future action. In cases like this, aims such as 'gain greater self-awareness' may suffice, and providing the therapist is very clear about the design of treatment (e.g. structure of activity), they can avoid vague treatment.

DESIGNING THE PROGRAMME

We now come to the third stage of planning treatment, namely designing the programme. Once the basic aims have been formulated, the more creative side of designing comes into play. Of course, the type of activities offered, and the method of structuring the programme, depends on each individual department's policy, and is clearly constrained by resources available. In general, however, designing a programme will involve manipulating and grading three dimensions in order to maximise therapeutic potential: the activity, the role of therapist, and the environment. Let us look in more depth at each of these in turn.

Activity

Central to occupational therapy, of course, is activity. As our primary tool we adapt and use activities purposefully to achieve our aims. These aims range from learning and practising skills to expressing and exploring emotions. We have a range of activities at our disposal spanning: individual treatments; large and small group work; work, social, domestic aspects; intellectual, physical, hobby interest, etc. The activities themselves are adapted and graded to increase or reduce demands on social, emotional, cognitive, perceptual or physical aspects. Activities are lengthened, shortened, made more complicated, spiced up with competition, rearranged for smaller groups, etc. The following chapter explores this area more fully.

The key consideration here is what aspects should be taken into account when deciding what activity to use in treatment. Basically five aspects need to be reviewed.

1. Aims of treatment — which activity can best fulfil the aims

of treatment, with scope for grading, whilst being appropriate for the patient (regarding their strengths, difficulties, age, gender and cultural appropriateness)?

2. Patient's choice — which activity is going to be most meaningful to the patient? 'The meaning of the activity, its choice, and satisfaction in it are determined by the individual patient's needs, interests, and motivations. They should not be determined by the occupational therapist's view of meaning' (Yerxa, 1979: 29). Whilst the therapist may set some of the parameters, she should offer choices to patients respecting their capacity to make their own decisions.

3. Therapist's choice — sometimes the patient is not able to choose which activity he or she would like to do (e.g. when acutely ill). The occupational therapist then chooses on the basis of her professional judgement and personal interest. Any therapist needs to have a degree of skill and interest in the chosen activity — at the very least a belief in the value of it (particularly important when dealing with patients who lack the necessary motivation).

4. Practical constraints — what activities are currently in operation, making the best use of existing resources? Limited funds may constrain opportunities to buy expensive equipment such as computers, kilns, etc. Limited staff resources may prevent certain activities running, e.g. lathework given safety factors. Limited resources can also be a source of inspiration, though, e.g. making 'rubbish collages', which can look very effective!

5. Balance of overall activity programme — it is important to consider the shape of the overall programme (e.g. week's timetable) and its total demands on the patient. Consider how best to balance the following to suit the individual: new and challenging or reassuring and safe; active or passive; diversional or emotionally charged; restful or stimulating; structure or freedom; staff-directed or patient-directed; abstract or concrete.

Role of therapist

A much-used, yet often-unexplored aim of treatment is 'establish rapport'. What exactly do we mean? It seems to be a phrase we use to acknowledge the fundamental importance of the relationship between patient and therapist. Often, as the therapist, it is our approach and the role we take with our patients which is the significant factor in the progress of treatment. We need to consider how best to encourage and motivate our patients, and make them feel safe. Does the patient respond best to our manner which is gentle or forceful? Humorous? Directive? Moreover, what role should we play? Consider the following range of possibilities: teacher, advice-giver, meeter of needs, model of normality, psychotherapist, behaviour-reinforcer, equipment-supplier, facilitator etc. Often, we adapt and modify our role as treatment progresses. In rehabilitation, for example, we grade our expectations by increasing the amount of autonomy and independence we give our patients, as we gradually reduce our support and direction, handing over responsibility.

The decision of what approach and role we take on can be determined by a range of factors. First and foremost the theoretical framework we are working within is, of course, a big influence. In the humanistic tradition we would incline towards being non-directive and accepting, encouraging creativity and self-expression. As a behaviourist we might be more directive in the way we reinforce behaviour and offer a structure for the patient. Secondly, the situation and activity is clearly a determinant of our approach. We are likely to be more directive if we need to manage a large group of patients, as opposed to one-to-one situations. Different activities also require different role-taking, such as being a 'teacher' when introducing a new task. The respective personalities involved also need considering. For example, a manner that works for one therapist could fail with another, simply because it comes across as artificial (a lesson here from counselling where 'genuineness' is seen as a core quality). Next, the team approach often guides our methods; for example when it decides a patient needs consistent handling or assigns a key worker to respond in a certain way (e.g. be confrontative). Finally, our approach has to mesh with colleagues with whom we may be working (i.e. co-therapists complementing each other). Here, one of the team may take a directive role controlling the group, while the other is supportive of individuals. In the times when staff shortages pre-empt such careful structuring, extra efforts should be made to guide nurses, students and helpers regarding how they could best contribute in an unfamiliar situation.

Theory into Practice
(Some guidelines for approaching different patients)

An anxious patient

Genuine reassurance given in a quiet, calm manner should be the main strategy used. Also valuable is our use of any 'relaxing', absorbing (thus diverting) activity, if the patient can be persuaded to join in. The key decision to make is whether or not the patient will benefit most from an undemanding or structured environment — the patient may appreciate being free to settle when ready, or may need the security of outside direction where the onus for any decision-making is removed.

A suspicious/deluded patient

Two main 'rules' apply here: (a) try to keep conversation (and activity) on a concrete, straightforward plane; (b) avoid getting locked into circular discussions, trying to reason the patient out of his or her beliefs. An initial clear explanation about the situation is important (e.g. 'The way I see it is . . .'), but it is unlikely to help to keep repeating your view. Diversionary tactics may work, such as 'before we talk more about that, can you try to concentrate on this activity for a few minutes?' Another possible strategy is to empathise with what is 'real', e.g. not responding to the patient's fear of 'outer space electricity', but responding to the fear.

A potentially suicidal patient

The highly emotive issue of potential suicide can only be handled if we take any threats seriously, and try to minimise our own value judgements (and advice as to why the patient should live). When faced with a patient expressing a wish to die, our best role is to listen and allow him or her to express the tensions which have lead to this point. Any suicidal patient should be carefully monitored by the team, with general precautions (e.g. not leaving the patient alone, removing scissors) being taken as necessary. We should not have the suicidal patient in activity groups unless we have adequate staff resources to give one-to-one attention if necessary.

A confused, disorientated patient

Reassurance, routine and structure are the important elements here. The patient's daily programme and environment should be well-organised and consistent. Devices such as written timetables and clear signposts are helpful, especially when combined with the human touch, where the therapist gently and clearly repeats basic information. As with any management strategy, it is most successful when applied consistently by the team.

A patient whose behaviour is uncontrolled/hyperactive

There are many strategies which might be tried, according to what the individual responds to best. Whilst ignoring the behaviour may help, the reverse can also be true (e.g. giving a little extra attention or reassuring physical contact may prevent the behaviour escalating). In any case, the therapist should give patients some feedback on what is difficult about the behaviour, and allow them the opportunity to take responsibility for controlling themselves. When the behaviour is so disturbed it disrupts the rest of a group, such a patient may need to be temporarily excluded (a one-to-one activity may be more appropriate at this stage anyway.) Activities requiring aggressive/gross motions may help to release some tensions, but often they also increase arousal, so should be used carefully.

An aggressive patient

Possibly the most difficult aspect of coping with verbal or physical aggression is our own reactions to violence and controlling them. In most circumstances the therapist needs to set and maintain clear, consistent limits of what is acceptable, and enforce them when necessary (telling the patient to leave the group). If there is no physical danger to anyone at stake (e.g. verbal abuse), the situation should be handled in a calm, matter-of-fact way designed to diffuse rather than provoke anger. If physical violence occurs, it needs to be dealt with immediately, so be clear about your unit's

71

policy/procedures. Whilst we must try to ensure the safety of all patients, we also have a right to keep ourselves free from physical harm. The team is an important support when any of us suffer from the understandable anxieties that occur, following a violent incident.

Environment

In therapy the environment consists of the human element of the people around and their attitudes, and the non-human aspects of the physical surroundings. These are manipulated in many subtle ways to achieve a range of goals. Firstly, the occupational therapy area needs to fit its purpose. Often it acts as an area where patients are expected to take on active and different roles, particularly if they have taken passive or sick roles elsewhere. If required, the environment also needs to be suited to the learning of new skills, which necessarily applies both to physical equipment and emotional support. Thus we manipulate our environment in terms of providing varied and selected stimulation to maximise learning and effective functioning. Here we darken rooms for relaxation, simulate industrial therapy workshops, provide free expression/graffiti walls and so on. We also carefully balance quiet spaces with active, more noisy sections. The options are endless and depend much on the needs of the patient group as well as available resources — the key is that we recognise its importance.

Secondly, a significant part of the environment consists of the people involved. Whether an activity takes place in a group or an individual setting is crucial. Choice of group size is itself important (six to eight patients or less if they are disturbed, is the usual small group number), and is often dependent on an assessment of how mutually supportive the group members are likely to be, or their developmental levels. The other human, though less tangible, aspect is the atmosphere and attitudes of people around. What 'feel' does the department have? Caring? Busy? Accepting? Do patients feel encouraged? If the answers are in the negative, is there anything that can be done to change the 'feel' in more positive directions?

Lastly, the physical environment in terms of type of room, comfort, arrangements of seating and positioning, layout of equipment, etc. are all very relevant aspects. Slight modifications in any of these can have dramatic effects on people's performance and attitudes (e.g. using floor cushions rather than chairs to promote an informal, relaxed atmosphere, or sitting a group around in a circle to promote interaction).

SUMMARY OF HOW TO PLAN TREATMENT

Organise information

1. Process all assessment information;
2. Identify problems in functional terms;
3. Identify strengths to build on;
4. Select priority problem/s.

Establish aims and goals

1. Establish overall aim;
2. Identify short- and long-term aims.
3. Set specific goals.

Design the programme, arranging:

1. Activity — the choice of which activity, and its demands, depends on aims, patient's preference, therapist's selection, practical constraints and overall programme balance. Consider how to grade the activity in order to achieve your aim; for example, increase complexity of task to facilitate higher learning of problem-solving skill.
2. Role of therapist — therapist's role includes the general approach to a patient and specific ways of handling behaviour, and the use of self/relationship as a therapeutic tool. It depends on the theoretical framework, situation, personalities involved, etc. Consider how to grade your role in order to achieve the desired aim; for example, become less directive and reduce support to encourage greater independence in the patient.
3. Environment — environment includes people involved and their attitudes and physical structures. Consider how to set up the environment in order to achieve your aim; for example,

reduce amount of tools available for use, to encourage sharing between people.

Theory into Practice
(Case example – planning treatment)

Background

Melanie, aged 30, has been in hospital for the past six years and is chronically disabled with schizophrenia. On moving her to a new rehabilitation ward the team aim to gradually resettle Melanie into a sheltered group home.

Current key problems

1. Institutionalised presentation and passive behaviour;
2. Poor task skills, i.e. she needs assistance to complete basic tasks;
3. Poor interpersonal skills, e.g. withdrawn, minimal group skills of sharing and awareness.

Overall treatment strategy

Short-term:
1. Reduce institutionalised behaviour;
2. Raise task skill ability;
3. Improve interpersonal skills (area chosen for occupational therapy intervention).

Middle-term:
1. Teach domestic and group skills relevant to group home;
2. Engage in community orientation programme.

Long-term:
   Gradually resettle in home with support continuing hospital attendance during the day.

Occupational therapy

Aims. To improve group interaction skills in particular, encourage verbal interaction with others, help to learn how to participate in a shared task and increase awareness of the presence and needs of others

---

Example goal. By taking a developmental approach, and using a variety of group activities, enable Melanie to move from interacting at a parallel level to participating comfortably in a project-level group.

Programme considerations

Session to run daily for two hours with one key therapist. Developmental approach treatment to commence on availability of a project-level group, consisting of three to six patients.

Activity

Provide a variety of relevant activities suitable for project group, such as cooking a meal. Grading: initially each member works alone on one aspect with assistance from therapist e.g. setting table, peeling potatoes. Later, members work together, e.g. wash and dry dishes, peel and chop vegetables; always eating the meal together at the end.

Therapist

1. Active, directive role, teacher of skills;
2. Major source of need satisfaction, encouraging trust;
3. Reinforces co-operative behaviour, encourages interaction;
4. Responsible for organising activity.

Grading: Gradually lessen one-to-one care and help, e.g. encourage group to make own decisions increasingly.

Environment

For example, kitchen: considering safety aspects and space, and ensuring appropriate equipment and supplies available. When possible, work as a group around a table to encourage members to acknowledge each other. Grading: gradually reduce supplies/equipment to encourage sharing, e.g. using only one pair of kitchen scales.

DISCUSSION QUESTIONS

1. Effective treatment cannot be planned without discussions with the team and with the patient. Discuss.
2. What should we do if a patient refuses to, or is unable to, participate in treatment planning?
3. What are the differences between aims, goals and objectives? Give examples, recognising the difference between therapy-centred and patient-centred goals.
4. The aim 'establish rapport' is unhelpful and too simplistic. Discuss.
5. What aspects of treatment are manipulated and graded, and how?
6. To what extent (and for whom) is it important to write down the treatment plan and programme?

5

Activity as Treatment

The belief in the healing power of activities has largely defined our profession over the years. Early pioneers emphasised how the health of individuals could be influenced by purposeful activities, by 'the use of muscles and mind together in games, exercise and handicraft, as well as in work' (Hopkins, 1983: 3). But what does activity offer, and why do we use it? When we say activity is purposeful and therapeutic what do we mean? Why do occupational therapists put so much store in 'doing', being active and involved?

This chapter seeks to demonstrate the ways in which the purposeful use of activity — namely the process of engaging in carefully structured activity, plus its end-result — is therapeutic. In this chapter I will explore the ways we use activity as treatment, by taking four different perspectives. Firstly I will consider the value of experiencing activity generally; I will then describe and evaluate some of the specific activities we offer in occupational therapy. Next our process of analysing activity to enable effective application will be examined, followed by three case illustrations of the use of activity in problem-solving.

THE VALUE OF ACTIVITY

Activity has value at many different levels, and we can see this applied both to therapy and to ourselves. We use it as a learning tool to help us explore ourselves, others and the environment. A child's use of activity, in the form of play, clearly illustrates how one can use it to practise/learn skills and to test out knowledge and perceptions. Activity also activates us. It motivates and energises us at a physical and mental level, stimulating the senses. Consider the times you have felt lethargic and sluggish, but after some exercise have then felt revitalised. The process of engaging in activity can be a form of play, and has its social value. It can be both pleasurable and diversional. At the very least it is something to do. At best we can have fun, be sociable and relate to others. Activity can be a vehicle to express and explore feelings, as in, for example, writing a diary. It can act projectively, release tensions, and even be cathartic. Further, both the process of, and the end-results of, activity have a work value, and can be gratifying, meeting needs of esteem, of being purposeful and creative or productive, whilst carrying with it tangible rewards. Linked with this area, activity promotes an awareness of our own capacity, a sense of competence and mastery, especially through success experience. And finally, many occupational therapists (e.g. those using the Model of Human Occupation system) would assert activity is fundamental to human existence as we have an innate, spontaneous tendency to be active, to explore our world. (see figure 5.1).

Figure 5.1: Values of activity

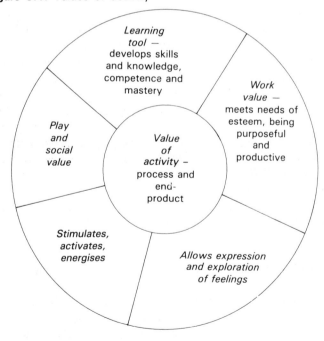

Behind any notion of the value of activity is an acknowledgement of how activity can potentially meet 'needs' at every level. This can be illustrated by using Maslow's 'hierarchy of needs' as a reference (Maslow, 1954). Cooking, for example, offers opportunities to satisfy: physiological needs, if a person is hungry; esteem needs, if he or she receives praise; mastery needs, as the individual learns new skills; and self-actualisation needs, if he or she simply enjoys cooking. Group work, as another example, can offer an individual the opportunity to have his or her love and belonging needs met when he or she is accepted by the group, as well as his or her esteem needs met, if he or she is recognised as having an important role.

Thus occupational therapists believe in activity for all its inherent values. They also however, place emphasis on activities being structured, adapted and graded purposefully. Here we analyse activities in order to understand their component parts and inherent demands, and then carefully apply the activity to suit an individual or group, to enhance their functioning. Generally occupational therapists modify, and therapeutically use, activities with five main aims in mind.

1. To help a patient acquire new skills, e.g. to help the patient cope better in the present, as seen in relaxation, or for the future, such as when we suggest a new hobby;
2. To improve specific areas of deficit, e.g. cognitive skills being improved with extra training of quizzes or work tasks;
3. To raise self-esteem of the patient, through he or she gaining confidence from any achievements, and gaining further awareness about his or her capacities and potential;
4. To provide an enjoyable, social outlet through activities spanning the range of both diversional and group-work experiences;
5. Lastly, we use activities to assess a patient's performance and measure any progress in the future.

A RANGE OF OCCUPATIONAL THERAPY ACTIVITIES

There are a vast number of activities at the disposal of occupational therapists, given that theoretically we can use any activity that is legal! Of course, this is constrained somewhat by what the patients want to do themselves, and the resources available. There are a number of activities which seem to turn up regularly in our repertoire, within occupational therapy programmes. Some of these will be briefly described and evaluated, to give a flavour of these aims and therapeutic use.

Figure 5.2: The therapy activities spectrum

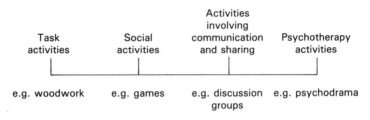

Occupational therapy activities are commonly described in terms of their content as pertaining to work, social, domestic or personal aspects of daily life. It is perhaps equally useful to describe the range of activities in terms of their basic aims and processes. In exploring this latter notion we can view activities along a spectrum, moving for the teaching of task skills to exploring feelings in psychotherapy (figure 5.2). Of course these divisions are not rigid as:

1. Most activities can be adapted to fit into one or other category depending on the desired aim. Art, for example, can be equally used as a work task or projectively.
2. Any one activity can simultaneously fit into several levels, e.g. a pottery work group may also be a social gathering.
3. Each individual will respond differently to an activity. Embroidery may be considered a relaxing social activity for a person skilled in it, but a rather daunting challenge for the uninitiated.

The following four sections examine these activity groupings in more detail. The descriptions offered are necessarily brief, but serve as examples showing the richness and variety of occupational therapy activities.

Task activities

These activities aim to improve skills — our daily living, work or task performance skills. They can be run at all levels, from trying to improve concentration in a craft group to work simulation and training.

Cookery

Cooking is a commonly used occupational therapy activity, mainly because it can be so easily graded whilst being almost universally practical. It offers opportunities for patients to develop task performance skills (e.g. following instructions, problem-solving), and can also be applied to later stages of treatment when patients are practising their domestic role skills (e.g. home management units using cookery as part of wider domestic rehabilitation). Cooking seems to be enjoyed by patients of all age groups and abilities, not least because of enjoyable end-products.

Industrial therapy

The widespread use of simulating factory workshops, offering assembly lines for packaging, etc., appears to be slowly diminishing. Certainly, any work rehabilitation in today's economic climate is problematic, and now usually geared towards improving work skills and offering a work role, than towards vocational resettlement. Care needs to be taken, when using industrial work, that therapeutic goals remain the prime target, as opposed to keeping people occupied, or using cheap labour, which are the common criticisms of industrial therapy. Certainly a well-run unit has much scope given the potential values of work in its widest sense.

Gardening

Horticulture is attracting many converts. Gardening offers much, as it can be graded from simple windowbox watering to taking responsibility for a vegetable plot in the long term. It provides opportunities to learn new hobby skills which can be realistically applied, for example, on discharge, as well as opportunities to nurture something which can grow and tangibly produce rewards.

Reality orientation

The specific use of work groups to treat problems of memory, confusion and disorientation can be commonly seen, particularly in units for the elderly. Here a classroom-type approach can be

81

Theory into Practice
(Example activity evaluation — *Pottery*)

Value
1. Improves task peformance skills, e.g. concentration, following instructions, attention to detail.
2. Easily graded for those with different skill levels, to ensure successful end-product.
3. Outlet for creativity and self-expression.
4. Offers tactile/sensory experience.
5. Hobby interest and leisure pursuit (e.g. night classes).
6. Used in graded programmes, e.g. for tolerance to dirt.

Ways of adapting
1. Length of process and patient involvement, e.g. from wedging to firing, or just making a pot.
2. Activity itself — thumb pots, coil pots, slab pots, decorative tiles, wheel, sculpture, group collage such as a village scene, etc.
3. Types of equipment — clay, Playdoh, plasticine, flour and water, or use of different tools and machinery.

Considerations
1. Messiness, e.g. for some it can be distressing.
2. Ensuring success versus not protecting patient from failure (make this decision for each individual).
3. Resources — can be expensive, a separate area may be required, a skill technician may be useful to 'make good' mistakes and offer high-level teaching/ideas.
4. Length of time for whole process, e.g. some people may find the wait for the glazed product difficult, and need more immediate results.

---

taken where basic information (e.g. of day, date, weather, names) is reiterated and reinforced, whilst a range of appropriate activities, e.g. memory games, are geared to maximising function. The most successful reality orientation remains that which is reinforced by the entire team, and recognises the individual patient's needs and dignity (a 24-hour approach). The body of reasearch into the effectiveness of this technique is increasing, with the bulk of evidence supporting the hypothesis that reality orientation is effective, particularly when used by the team to combat confusion. Evidence concerning the value of memory activities is mixed. (For more in-depth discussions on research and applications see Holden and Woods, 1988.)

Social activities

The wide spectrum of social activities are primarily aimed at promoting enjoyment and leisure interest. They can be used at a simple level as diversion, and upwards, to more purposeful ends involving social contact and interaction.

Crafts

The range of crafts, from traditional activities such as basketry to more recently introduced activities such as photography, offer much for every age group and ability level. A group of patients sitting in a circle, engaged in a craft, is a common sight in many departments. These activities are both useful for task skills, and provide a focal point for social interaction. The most successful craft departments seem to be those where clear aims are pursued and products are attractively displayed or sold (as opposed to being thrown away or re-used).

Sports

The trend for healthy physical activities, from jogging to aerobics, has also been reflected in occupational therapy departments. A range of activities can be encompassed here, from gym exercises to team sports such as volley ball. The competitive and non-competitive games offer enjoyment as well as opportunities for challenge and group interaction.

Indoor games

This range encompasses drama-type games (e.g. charades), quizzes (e.g. general knowledge), board games (e.g. Trivial Pursuits), and group activities such as bingo. Again the way the activities are structured greatly varies the end-results. Bingo, for example, can be used as a way of teaching number/letter recognition, or to encourage interaction (e.g. if patients share a card), or simply for fun.

Theory into Practice
(Example activity evaluation — *Dance*)

Value
1. Enjoyable/fun.
2. Socialising value of mixing with others (and possibly touching).
3. Promotes awareness of body movement and posture.
4. Stimulating, activating.
5. Can promote health, circulation, physical well-being, etc.
6. Sensory integration programmes.
7. Easily graded to suit any age group and skill level.

Ways of adapting
1. Activity itself — aerobics, old-time dance, jazz dance, disco dance, movement to music, Medau, mirroring, etc.
2. Complexity of steps.
3. Individual, partnership or group dancing.
4. New learning versus old skills.

Considerations
1. Resources — often need a skilled/experienced teacher.
2. Health risk, e.g. overexertion in aerobics or contra-indications for heart/lung problems.
3. Special clothes/shoes required.
4. People may be overly conscious of their body shape, or have problems in touching others/being touched.

Reminiscence therapy

In contrast to reality orientation, reminiscence therapy offers patients the opportunity to share old memories and discuss how times have changed. A range of slides, pictures and equipment are available for use, with the precaution of ensuring the patients are brought back to the present day at the end of the session. A useful textbook for reference covering this area is Coleman (1986).

Activities involving communication and sharing

These aspects can be incorporated into almost any activity, though most often fall under the guise of 'group work'. Group members are encouraged to share their experiences and provide mutual support and encouragement. Often the format of the activity is determined by the theoretical framework used (as seen when comparing dramatherapy and social skills training).

Discussion groups

These are handled in many ways, adapting aims, structure/format and the therapist role. At one level, for example, we can have a 'hat discussion' (hat containing topic suggestions on slips of paper) to formalise discussions. At another level more personal sharing can be promoted by, for example, reading out and discussing the problem page/Agony Aunt letters in magazines.

Dramatherapy

This term encompasses remedial drama, socio-drama, role-play, psychodrama, and contains a wide range of activities, including games, action scenarios and group communication exercises (Jennings, 1987). From its essentially humanistic base it can offer much to any age group and ability level, providing it is well handled. Some exercises may seem 'threatening' or 'childish' with inhibitions and resistances from group members, preventing movement. If taken slowly, however, and at a suitable level, the dramatherapy slot in the programme, with its emphasis on 'play', 'acting out' and group processes, can be the central pivot of therapy.

Social skills training

This technique is sometimes confused with general skills education with the mentally handicapped, or with dramatherapy. In its purest use, however, it is designed as a behavioural technique; to teach, systematically, elements of social behaviour (verbal, non-verbal, assertion, etc.). Patients who benefit may never have acquired the skills (e.g. mentally handicapped people), or had the skills once and lost them (e.g. institutionalised patients), or have the skills but lack the confidence to apply them (e.g. anxious patients). Its practical emphasis on 'doing' and step-by-step learning of skills via role play, modelling, feedback, etc. make it a particularly relevant technique to use in occupational therapy.

Theory into Practice
(Example activity evaluation — *'Trust Games'*)

Value
1. Group cohesion and working together.
2. Relaxing and pleasant sensations.
3. Trusting others physically promotes emotional trust.
4. Physical risk-taking promotes emotional risk-taking
5. Enjoyable/fun.

Ways of adapting
1. Activity itself — group lifts, swaying in a circle, fall-backs, run 'n' jump, blind walks, robots, etc.
2. Amount of risk and/or support.
3. Partnerships and different groupings.

Considerations
1. Physical safety — e.g. strained backs are common with poor lifting techniques. Careful instructions are necessary, plus accurate calculations of numbers of people needed.
2. Emotional safety — e.g. patient may be dropped or not handled sensitively. Whilst this may not be physically damaging, a sense of trust will not be developed. The therapist needs to feel that the group members will handle each other gently. She may need to step in and more directively take control in order to pre-empt any insensitive handling.
3. Contracts can be useful, e.g. (a) being 'responsible for your own body', or (b) not forcing anyone.
4. Correct clothing important.
5. Some members may be overly conscious of their weight or body, or have inhibitions about touch.

Special sensitivity is needed, however, to tread the line between imposing one's own standards of behaviour and facilitating the development of new or different behaviours in someone who wants to change. Two useful texts in this area are Argyle (1981) and Ellis and Whittington (1981).

Psychotherapy activities

These highly specialised activities arise mainly from the psychodynamic school, and focus on facilitating the expression and exploration of feelings. The activities can be more analytically based, emphasising unconscious conflict and symbols, or

---

Theory into Practice
(Example activity evaluation — *Projective Art*)

Value

Note two different stages of: 'doing it' (the art process itself of, for example, painting a picture) and 'talking about it' afterwards (discussion or psychotherapy; for example 'what I am trying to say in this picture is . . .')

1. Self-awareness, insight.
2. Expression and exploration of emotions or catharsis.
3. Group communication, sharing, cohesion, support.
4. Enjoyable.

Ways of adapting

1. Extend the time for either 'doing' or 'talking'
2. Activity itself — free self-expression, fun games, painting to music, painting to a theme, interpretive analysis, etc.
3. Vary themes and titles, e.g. 'How I see myself now . . . in five years', 'my family', 'schizophrenia', 'happiness', What I like/dislike', 'what alcohol means to me . . .'
4. Media used — clay, paint, fingerpaint, collage, rollerbrushes, etc.

Considerations

1. Emotional safety/trust within the group essential.
2. Emphasise the importance of free spontaneous art as opposed to being concerned about artistic end-product.
3. Contraindications: (a) dangers of stirring up feelings as activity can be emotionally powerful; (b) over-interpretation can be offensive or simply wrong; (c) may reinforce fantasy, confusion, with, e.g., those with thought disorder.

---

more humanistic where self-awareness and growth are the end goals.

Psychodrama

This dramatic technique, pioneered by Moreno, can be a powerful tool. Individuals enact/re-enact life scenes in an effort to explore their emotions, unconscious needs and relationships, both real and fantasy. Specific techniques are utilised, such as role play and role reversal, using the 'empty chair', and 'soliloquy'. Like all psychotherapy, skill, experience and some training is necessary before taking on a leader/director role.

Non-directive play therapy

This technique, pioneered by Virginia Axline (1971), has been used as a model for many occupational therapists working in child psychiatry. Briefly, a child is offered the free use of a playroom, to play out feelings, needs and fantasies. The therapist attempts to be non-judgemental, and lets the child lead, acting mainly as a mirror to reflect back the play's content to the child.

ACTIVITY ANALYSIS

One of the key skills of an occupational therapist is her ability to analyse the component parts of an activity in order to use it purposefully, enhancing a patient's growth and functioning. Whilst the step-by-step analysis can feel a laborious process it is essential, until the therapist feels familiar with both the nature of the activity and its potential as a treatment medium.

What do we analyse?

Basically, we view the activity at all levels investigating:

1. the steps, procedures and processes involved
2. materials and tools required
3. motions and sequences involved
4. the social and environmental context
5. the results of the process.

We look at these aspects, paying particular attention to how demanding the activity is in terms of a person's functioning in the following areas:

Physical — e.g. what type of movements are required: fine? gross? repetitive? aggressive? What kind of tolerance and strength is needed?

Sensory/perceptual — e.g. what visual, tactile, proprioceptive aspects are involved?

Cognitive — e.g. how much concentration, memory, intellectual ability, abstract thought, etc., is needed?

Emotional — e.g. does the activity ease expression of feelings? Does it satisfy needs? Is it stimulating? Is it intrinsically/extrinsically motivating?

Social — e.g. what level of communication skill is required? How much sharing and co-operative behavior is expected?

In addition to analysing the demands of the activity on the patient, other demands, may be noted, such as: 'this activity needs attention paid to detail', or 'some amount of tolerance to dirt is required', or 'there are cultural assumptions behind this activity making it unsuitable for certain groups'. Thus we build up a picture of the inherent nature of the activity and its demands. We then marry this information with the individual patient's needs, ability and motivation.

Why analyse an activity?

Having broken down an activity into its steps and demands, we can utilise the activity's potential to restore/maintain function. This can be seen clearly in four ways:

1. We analyse an activity to determine if a patient can do it. For example, the apparently simple task of making a collage may not be so easily achieved if it takes place in a group setting, and the patient involved is operating below a parallel group level (See Chapter 2 — Mosey's group interaction skill). Or as another example we might feel more confident about encouraging a patient to use a pottery wheel if we assess he or she has sufficient standing tolerance, co-ordination, as well as familarity with claywork and

89

some perseverance while learning a new skill. (Note that if the occupational therapist is trying to promote growth/increase skill levels, some aspect of the activity should be slightly beyond the patient's ability, creating a goal to strive for.)

2. We also may break down an activity into smaller steps and subtasks, for teaching purposes. An accurate preliminary analysis allows us to consider if there is a logical progression or if any steps need to be simplified or eliminated. The process of teaching someone how to make a coil pot, for example, might involve a step-by-step progression of:

   a) therapist demonstrates showing basic idea and result
   b) patient makes base after another demonstration and with physical and verbal promoting
   c) patient practises making coils with advice
   d) patient makes coils and applies to pot using slip, after instruction and demonstration
   e) patient shown how to finish off coil pot
   f) patient makes another pot with minimal instruction given.

   Each stage of the process contains its own skill levels and needs to be carried out in sequence if the end-product is to be successful. Throughout the teaching it is also important to consider the patient's cognitive ability as well as his or her needs for reward or encouragement.

3. We also analyse activities in order to identify what aspects need to be adapted or altered, in order to ensure a useful experience suited to the patient's functional ability. Thus the patient who finds working in a group difficult, and is unable to join in a group collage, may be asked to make an individual collage which is later added to the larger one. Or the patient learning to cook, who is unable to read, may need picture recipe cards instead of written ones.

4. Lastly, we analyse activity in order to grade it appropriately to bring about change. We can identify which components need to be made more demanding, thereby stretching function. An example of this can be seen in woodwork, where treatment might move from simple sanding to making intricate sculpture puzzles, encouraging the patient daily towards higher amounts of concentration or attention to detail.

ACTIVITY AND PROBLEM-SOLVING

One mistake occupational therapists can make, in using activities, arises when we feel confident about the value of an activity, and thus assume its therapeutic effect. An example of this is the patient who has the problem of poor eye contact, and is encouraged to play a game of 'wink-murder' because it utilises eye contact. Another patient, with poor concentration, is given dressmaking, as it requires some mental application. On careful examination, though, it is clear these activities will only prove beneficial as part of a graded programme. Thus, wink murder is only useful (for eye contact) if a patient finds it slightly difficult to do, and this requires the occupational therapist to carefully adjust the demands of the game. Likewise, the patients with poor concentration who engage in dressmaking, will need regular encouragement by the occupational therapist, enabling them to attend to the task. It is not the dressmaking itself which improves concentration, but how it is applied.

Let us consider three examples of how activities can be applied as part of the problem-solving process. Primarily we achieve this by modifying and grading the activity itself. The examples also show how both the therapist's approach and her structuring of the environment, are fundamentally linked to the grading of an activity.

Case example No. 1

Problem: poor task performance skills.
Activity: woodwork.
Grading: increasing the demands and complexity of task.

Michael, aged 40, had had repeated admissions to hospital with a diagnosis of schizophrenia. His basic task performance was poor, probably resulting from a combination of cognitive deficit stemming from his illness, passive behaviour due to institutionalisation, and the sedating effects of his medication. A concrete task for which Michael expressed an interest, was woodwork.

Stage 1: Basic task and quick results

With his concentration being so poor initially, the occupational therapist encouraged Michael to make something which could be

91

completed fairly quickly, and that required a minimal amount of
skill. Over the first week several tasks were completed, such as
varnishing a ready-made stool, and sanding and polishing a bread-
board for the ward. These activities required the minimum of
instruction, and were repetitive enough to allow Michael's attention to wander, whilst still producing constructive end-products.

Stage 2: Increased task demands

As Michael settled into the routines of the new area, more
complex tasks were introduced involving more complex instructions, and which took longer amounts of time. He first made a
plant trough out of already cut strips of wood, which he then
painted. Later, with the occupational therapist's help, he made an
intricate chessboard requiring careful staining and varnishing of
the wood.

Case example No. 2

Problem: lack of self-confidence.
Activity: jewellery making with metalwork.
Grading: early success experience leading on to increased task
demands and difficulties as therapist gradually reduces supportive
assistance.

> (*Discussion point*. Lack of confidence is a problem that most
> of us have in some area or other, and it is usually situation-
> specific. Activity, and 'doing' treatments, can only problem-
> solve successfully if the confidence problem involves ability to
> do/achieve. At its most basic level, though, any quick, tangible
> success experience is likely to result in some positive self-
> feelings. If the experience is too easy then negative feelings
> can be confirmed, which brings into play the use of careful
> grading. At a deeper level problem-solving confidence is likely
> to only work over a longer term, and will entail a judicious
> mixture of appropriate therapist handling and grading of
> activity.)

June, a 23-year-old, unemployed woman, greatly lacked confidence in her abilities. She had started several college courses,
but either failed or gave up. She felt 'useless', but agreed to give
occupational therapy a chance.

Stage 1: Introducing the activity

June expressed an interest in jewellery making, though also said 'I won't be able to make anything as nice as those samples'. The occupational therapist suggested she give it a week, and that she first learn the basic skills. This approach was adopted to avoid being overly praising, as June was likely to negate compliments or reassurances, and also to encourage June to be more realistic about her skills.

Stage 2: Teach basic skills and provide success experience

The occupational therapist taught June a simple and quick method of beading and bending a piece of wire to make an earring. June was provided with a range of examples and ideas, and was encouraged to 'have a go'. The results were successful, came quickly, and provided an immediate reward. June could not deny she could produce some basic, pretty jewellery.

Stage 3: Increase demands of activity

After June's initial good feelings about her achievement died down she began to put down her skill, saying the task was too easy. The occupational therapist agreed, and showed her a much more complicated method requiring new welding and enamelling techniques. The occupational therapist supervised and encouraged June more carefully, initially trying to pre-empt failure.

Stage 4: Reduce therapist support

As June's ability and confidence grew, the occupational therapist withdrew both her help and encouragement. The occupational therapist began to 'allow' June to use her own ideas, and make mistakes, and also more realistically gave constructive criticisms. Thus June could feel unqualified confidence from her results.

Case example No. 3

Problem: inability to share — group interaction skills.
Activity: collage.
Grading: amount of sharing required increased.
(Treatment notes: This problem of inability to share can be seen within a developmental frame of reference, e.g. Mosey's parallel/project group levels. As such, treatment is systematically geared towards being a learning process which involves modifying the

activity, the environment and the therapist's role. As Mosey states, a patient should be placed in a group which demands slightly more than he or she feels comfortable with, if learning is to take place. In this example an already existing 'project group' is established, consisting of seven other patients who are at early project level. The group would meet daily for an hour to engage in a mixture of activities, e.g. collage.) Willis, aged 26, has suffered from a manic-depressive illness which results in him being self-absorbed and occasionally infantile in his behaviour. One main problem is his difficulty in group interaction, which resulted in his referral to the Project Group.

Stage 1: Early-level project group experience

Willis is introduced to the group and joins their activity, which takes place around one table. Each patient is asked to make his or her own individual collage, from cutting out pictures of food from magazines and sticking them onto a sheet of paper. At the end the occupational therapist encourages the group members to be aware of each other and work together more, by asking them to arrange each individual's sheet with the others', on a larger poster. Willis found the latter task of working with the whole group more difficult, so he remained more passive.

Stage 2: Medium-level project group experience

After a few sessions similar to the above, the occupational therapist encourages Willis and the others to make a collage in pairs, requiring them to minimally share and interact with at least one other person. Willis enjoyed this, and was also able to work a bit with the group as a whole, as they discussed how to arrange the pictures.

Stage 3: Advanced-level project group experience

On a later occasion the occupational therapist encouraged the group to make a collage as a whole. Individuals first collected their own pile of 'rubbish', such as leaves or empty matchboxes. These were then placed all together in a pile. The group then stuck the bits randomly onto a large card. Willis was given the responsibility at the end to spray the collage an attractive gold colour. At this level of group working the therapist attempted to further group sharing and awareness of others, by promoting discussion and also by reducing the amount of glue and scissors available.

*　　*　　*

In all, we use a variety of activities in occupational therapy, and in order to effectively apply them we need to appreciate their specific properties and limitations. The therapeutic potential of an activity mainly emerges when it is carefully structured and graded for the individuals concerned. Thus our belief in the healing power of activities comes both from its intrinsic value and from the way it is applied.

The only question that remains to be asked is the extent to which only activity is fundamental to occupational therapy? How much scope does that leave for us to get involved in other aspects? There is an ongoing debate, for example, about whether the use of counselling (consisting more of talking rather than doing) is a legitimate tool for occupational therapists. Some would say it is not true occupational therapy, and merely an example of our jumping on a fashionable bandwagon and the trend towards role-blurring with other team members. Others would say it is an important part of our problem-solving process, and providing that occupational therapy concerns (e.g. of role performance, time structuring) are the focus, then counselling, is a legitimate function. In addition, activity is simply one key therapy tool, as the use of ourselves and structuring the environment are of equal importance in occupational therapy. This debate is currently a central one, and it refers to questions about our role and where we are going. It began with a move away from arts and crafts into industrial work, creative and behavioural therapies. Now talking therapies such as counselling are being scrutinised. The key to the debate is about whether or not we want to unify and limit our profession to activity only. What do you think?

DISCUSSION QUESTIONS

1. The therapeutic value of occupational therapy activities arises from the grading process rather than any inherent value of the activity itself. Discuss.
2. What aspects of an activity need to be analysed, and why?
3. How can woodwork (or another activity) be graded to improve (a) task performance skills, (b) social interaction skills.
4. Work rehabilitation is irrelevant in today's economic climate.

Discuss.

5. What are the similarities and differences between dramatherapy and social skills training?

6. The use of counselling in occupational therapy goes against our role as it does not have an activity base. Discuss.

6

Implementation of Treatment

Any discussion on the implementation of treatment must seek to synthesise together all aspects of the occupational therapy process from assessment to evaluation, discussed in previous chapters. I have attempted to achieve this synthesis via an outline of eight contrasting case studies, chosen to illustrate the diversity of our therapy process. Each case study is intended to indicate both the different types of patients we treat, and our different treatment approaches. Though these case studies are not verbatim accounts of actual patients' records the material for them is drawn largely from my clinical experience, and so reflects the kinds of problems and treatments encountered in occupational therapy. In these examples I have tried to demonstrate some facts of occupational therapy, namely: our wide eclectic base; short- and long-term aspects of treatment; and some of the issues/complexities that can arise. The examples are necessarily selective guides to the scope and depth of our work, but I hope they will generate ideas for practice and discussion. For instance, if you disagree with the treatment described, what would you offer? Why?

In this chapter I have not produced discussion questions at the end. In place of these, as you go through each case study, reflect on the following questions:

1. What is the key occupational therapy role identifiable in each study, and what theoretical framework underpins each described treatment?
2. Select an alternative theoretical framework. How would this change the treatment applied?
3. In your view, how should the problems identified in each study be prioritised and handled?

4. How could the occupational therapist grade each suggested activity to effectively meet the associated aims?
5. How would each case study person be treated in your clinical set-up? Why?
6. Review the range of occupational therapy practice described in the case studies as a whole. Is there an underlying role common to all?

CASE STUDY 1 — SALLY, 32 YEARS OLD

Key issues: anxiety management and return to work.

Summary of history

Sally is admitted to an acute admission unit with a diagnosis of anxiety neurosis. She says she cannot cope any more with her panic attacks and tension headaches. She has even blacked out once, apparently from stress, during her work as a stylist in a hairdressing salon. She has a longstanding relationship with a man with whom she lives, and she appears to be experiencing tensions in this area as well.

Team strategy

On the ward she is given both medication (minor tranquillisers) and opportunities to express her feelings. The social worker becomes involved in doing some 'marital' counselling. The psychologists and occupational therapist work jointly to organise an anxiety-management programme.

Initial occupational therapy assessment

On interview she presents as being well-dressed and groomed, though anxious about her looks, as she keeps apologising for her tearful blotchy face and the fact that she has not put on any make-up. She stresses that she is particularly concerned that her panic attacks have been interfering with her work. Over the previous few months she has grown increasingly anxious that she was making mistakes and is being criticised for them. As a result, Sally was checking clients' hair excessively and this has resulted in their loss of confidence in her.

Treatment planning

What	How
1. Teach anxiety-management strategies	Anxiety-management course covering: (a) educational aspects of the nature of anxiety and cognitive restructuring (e.g. 'I *can* cope'); (b) relaxation and yoga classes; (c) group discussions on anxiety-coping strategies; (d) some music activities used for relaxation.
2. Raise her confidence to make her feel able to cope with her anxiety	
3. In the long term, facilitate her return to work (where she applies her new coping strategies)	Initially build her confidence by letting her do hair on the ward in a beauty care group. Later implement a graded return to work with some limited follow-up and supportive counselling

Progress of treatment

Sally was treated as an in-patient for one week, and as a day-patient for a further month. In the latter period she made a successful reintegration into her work, aided by supportive colleagues. The social worker continued to see Sally and her partner, as more fundamental problems seemed situated there. From the occupational therapy point of view, Sally gained much from the practical anxiety-management input and the support she gained from other group members.

Discussion

Sally's treatment can be approached from the perspectives of both humanistic values and behaviourism. On one hand we have the humanistic focus on Sally's lack of confidence in herself. Here, occupational therapy activities are applied to raise her esteem with success experience (beauty care), and give her a sense of control over her ability to cope (relaxation). On the other hand, the teaching of relaxation skills and the application of techniques such as cognitive restructuring and anxiety-management, stems more from the behavioural tradition. This two-pronged eclectic approach is continued when Sally is gradually returned to work. As occupational therapists we are concerned with her optimum functioning whilst carrying out her work role. The tools we use to get her there may be framed in a number of contrasting theories.

CASE STUDY 2 — GEORGE, 42 YEARS OLD

Key issues: chronic schizophrenia and rehabilitation.

Summary of history

George is attending a day hospital for long-term rehabilitation and support. He had his first schizophrenic breakdown when he was in his 20s and since then has spent a significant proportion of his life in the local hospital. Whilst maintained on long-term medication, his behaviour and skills show evidence of institutionalisation. His referral to the day hospital is an attempt to maintain his skills and life in the community, prevent in-patient admission, and provide him with some 'role' during the day. He lives with his sister (and her family) who also require some support and a break from George in the day.

Team strategy

The doctor monitors the medication and involves the family in some family therapy. The community psychiatric nurse undertakes regular home visits to monitor George and provide medication, and give the family support. The psychologist is involved in setting up a range of behaviour programmes including social skills training and token economy. The occupational therapist's concern is with George's skills (self-care, task performance and social).

Initial occupational therapy assessment

The priority problems identified, from observing George in activities and carrying out the standardised REHAB assessment (see Chapter 3), include:

1. Task performance — George's skills are poor; namely: poor concentration (less than ten minutes on routine work task), limited problem-solving ability, difficulty in following verbal instructions and lack of attention to detail.
2. General behaviour — compliance, dependence and passivity in evidence. Social skills reduced, especially his ability to initiate conversation, and posture and eye contact difficulties.
3. On the strengths side, George is friendly when approached and his self-care presentation is relatively good. This is likely to be due in part to his sister's influence.

He is also motivated to attend the day hospital and responds positively to both praise and concrete rewards such as tokens.

Treatment planning

What	How
1. Provide a work role to increase esteem/status and improve task performance skills	Light industrial work, grading, amount of concen tration required, respon- sibility, etc. Consider for the long term the possibility of sheltered work or day centre
2. Encourage sense of self, initiative, autonomy and responsibility	(a) Day hospital environment and consistent team approach; (b) success

What	How
	experience in work; (c) use of own behavioural target setting (e.g. 'by the end of the week I will have achieved . . .'); (d) investigations into his home/domestic work role aiming to increase input, in the long term.
3. Improve social skills and widen opportunities	(a) Once-weekly social skills group; (b) twice-weekly general social activities group within day hospital; (c) encouragement to take, for example, evening activities and holidays, both with family and outside.

Progress of treatment

George regularly attended the day hospital over a period of two years, when he eventually moved on to a local day centre (with the community psychiatric nurse maintaining contact. In the first year, treatment was geared to improving specific task skills in the industrial therapy workshop. The fortnightly self and supervisor appraisal and goal-setting interview (behavioural emphasis) was a significant part of his progress. He was promoted in his work position, which did much for his self-esteem. The latter part of George's rehabilitation focused on his involvement and role at home (trying to increase his level of responsibility taken), and a graded discharge to the day centre. George made some significant gains during his stay at the hospital, but remained vulnerable, needing a sheltered, structured environment.

Discussion

Any discussion of George's rehabilitation must include a recognition of the team approach found characteristically in many day hospitals. In these instances it is often difficult to identify a special occupational therapy role — indeed, we may sometimes feel confused when we see nurses managing industrial therapy units, or the psychologists running the social skills group! This poses the question of whether or not this is beneficial to the patients. Most team enthusiasts would say we should not defensively guard our role, but work together, drawing on our own particular skills.

Whilst role-blurring is an increasingly common phenomenon, the occupational therapist's specific role can still be understood in terms of the focus on the patient's work, social or domestic performance. In some units the occupational therapist may emphasise work roles and use industrial/clerical work. If the occupational therapists favour a more domestic line, they may use a half-way house or stress home management activities. Many of the more socially orientated therapists will explore the use of leisure and community facilities. All of these are a legitimate use of our time and skills — and given how important we think these aspects are, is it surprising that other professionals agree?

CASE STUDY 3 — MRS BROWN, 70 YEARS OLD

Key issues: bereavement, family and community support.

Summary of history

Mrs Brown has deteriorated markedly over the previous year since the death of her husband. She has neglected herself physically, being both depressed and forgetful. Living alone, she has become increasingly dependent on her married daughter who lives nearby. The daughter is concerned about her mother's poor self-care, safety and isolation, and has sought help from the general practitioner.

Team strategy

The general practitioner does a preliminary assessment on Mrs Brown and refers her to the community psychiatric team. On discussion, they decide that the occupational therapist should become the key worker, given her skills in both practical assessments and counselling, using back-up services as necessary (e.g. social worker to organise financial aspects and practical services). The team are concerned to assess Mrs Brown's exact level of functioning in her home, and to consider the future possibilities.

Initial occupational therapy assessment

Two home visits are undertaken. The first aims to establish initial contact with Mrs Brown and her daughter, the second focuses on Mrs Brown individually. Methods used are interview and observation. Key findings include observing problem areas of:

1. Skills — e.g. physically slow and absent-minded when making tea, looks slightly dishevelled, tends to neglect feeding herself.
2. Feelings — e.g. tearful when talking about husband, says she does not want to do anything except sit.
3. Behaviour — e.g. dependent on daughter, less capable/more feeble when daughter is around.
4. *Social* — e.g. isolated, little social contact except daughter's input.

The *positive aspects* which are identified include:

1. The fact that Mrs Brown's activities of daily living skills seem safe and intact, providing she concentrates on the task;
2. The daughter's willingness to be supportive;
3. The comfortable semi-detached bungalow which Mrs Brown owns and loves.

Treatment planning

What	How
1. Provide emotional support (considering her self-neglect within this)	Three days a week at the day hospital offering: (a) craft groups for social aspects; (b) cooking group to assess practical skills; (c) individual support/bereavement counselling.
2. Further assess domestic and self-care skills (to ensure safety)	
3. Work with mother/daughter relationship	A few joint sessions to negotiate mutual roles and time given by daughter, considering their individual needs
4. Widen social opportunities (providing her with outside involvements and interests)	Encourage Mrs Brown to join social clubs or do some voluntary work, etc.; day centre may be possibility.

Progress of treatment

Mrs Brown was initially reluctant to go to the day hospital, feeling both apathetic and uncertain about new life changes. She was persuaded to go for a trial period when her daughter agreed to drop and collect her by car. Once she settled into the day hospital she enjoyed the social contact and re-learned some old craft hobbies. The occupational therapist also saw Mrs Brown regularly on a one-to-one basis, offering support and allowing her to express feelings of her loss. The cooking sessions exposed some potential problems as Mrs Brown was occasionally unsafe, remaining slightly forgetful and confused, and in any case was not motivated to cook for herself. The issue of Mrs Brown's potential self-neglect regarding feeding herself, and her daughter's subsequent 'over-involvement', became the focus of treatment. A contract was established where Mrs Brown received lunch via meals-on-wheels or the day hospital, whilst she provided her own cold snacks in the morning and evening. Instead of cooking regularly for her mother, the daughter was encouraged to invite her to Sunday lunch with with family. In the long term Mrs Brown enjoyed going regularly to a new day centre. The occupational therapist continued to monitor her situation by visiting every few months.

Discussion

The domiciliary role played by this occupational therapist may strike you as a less common reflection of our occupational therapy role. However, our community input, working one-to-one (or with families) in their homes, is an increasing one, given the larger trends in this direction. Moreover, these interventions are often accompanied by a more manager-like function, where we refer the client on to other agencies (subject to availability). The question we need to ask is: 'Is this the direction we want to move in?' On the negative side it could be said we are encroaching on the social worker/ community psychiatric nurse roles, and are moving too far from our activity base. On the positive side we could say that, as occupational therapists, we are concerned to preserve a person's individuality and health, and these (in current thinking) are best achieved within the person's home. Further, whilst activity may not be the main therapeutic medium used, counselling about a person's daily life role/patterns is also central to occupational therapy.

CASE STUDY 4 — KEVIN, EIGHT YEARS OLD

Key issues: development of playskills and play therapy.

Summary of history

Kevin has been referred to a child psychiatry day unit after being suspended from school for his antisocial behaviour. He has a history of behaviour problems and bullying other children. Kevin was seen to have a close relationship with his mother, who tends to overprotect and cosset him, occasionally limiting his social contact with other children. This was due, in part, to Kevin's history of epilepsy, now controlled by drugs.

Team strategy

Each team member is given a specific role to play within the multi-disciplinary teamwork: the nurses and unit teachers work on Kevin's social interaction/behaviour; the psychologist investigates his cognitive functioning; the social worker engages the parents in family therapy; the occupational therapist acts as a play therapist.

Initial occupational therapy assessment

The occupational therapist initially attempts to use non-directive play with Kevin, offering 'free play' and a non-judgemental approach. This proves unworkable, however, as Kevin seems unable to play, and resorts to requesting structured, competitive board games. The occupational therapist decides to work more directively using play. Through puppets, painting and dressing-up activities, Kevin reveals his lack of imaginative/fantasy play (i.e. developmentally he seems to have missed out the play stage between three and seven years). Further, when uncertain about what to do next, he often becomes aggressive or demands to play a competitive game saying 'I'm going to win!' The occupational therapist hypothesises that a key problem for Kevin is his limited play skills, which in turn severely affect his peer interactions. On the strength side he is bright, with many other abilities (e.g. school work) and also he wants to make friends with others (but has never been able to).

Treatment planning

What	How
1. Establish a relationship with Kevin (making it 'safe' for him to lose occasionally or feel inadequate, as well as boosting his esteem)	Twice-weekly individual sessions with the occupational therapist taking a positive and encouraging attitude, whilst confronting him about his difficulties

What	How
2. Teach how to 'play' — encouraging flexibility, having fun and using imagination	Grade each activity for it's imagination level, acting first as a model
3. Lessen intensity for winning competitive games	Discuss issues of winning and losing, trying to practise handling the latter

Progress of treatment

A contract was first established where Kevin could choose any activity he wanted to do for the last ten minutes of the session, providing he joined in the occupational therapist's set activities earlier. The therapist invented a structured, competitive game which eventually could act as fantasy play. On trying to work constructively with Kevin's aggression she devised a competition of 'knocking down toy soldiers in the sandpit by throwing small plastic balls'. Kevin enjoyed this and it became his 'choice game' as well. The therapist approached the game encouraging the fun element, by using laughter and playing little games within, like 'throwing all the balls in one go, really quickly'. When the intensity for winning was reduced in Kevin, and he simply enjoyed his sessions, the occupational therapist increasingly added the element of imagination, e.g. speculating on what a soldier was thinking or felt like. The natural progression became more focus on the sandpit playing with the soldiers, having them fight and help each other, building barriers, inventing scenarios, etc. When Kevin was thoroughly familiar with this play other children were invited in for short periods to join in 'Kevin's game', which they all found great fun.

Discussion

Kevin's treatment clearly lies within a developmental framework of teaching skills. In common with all treatments we offer, alternative methods based on other theoretical frameworks are possible. Kevin's problem may well have been seen as a behavioural one (as the nurse prioritised) with his aggression to peers being targeted as the priority area for treatment. Here, behaviour modification using star charts and modelling could have been incorporated into a group activities programme. The humanistic occupational therapist, following the Axline approach, may have diagnosed an unhappy, lonely child, who needed to explore his feelings within an accepting relationship. The decision of which approach to take was largely organised according to the team's negotiation in an attempt to balance interventions. To some extent trial-and-error also had a part to play (e.g. the initial unsuccessful use of free play).

CASE STUDY 5 — PHILLIP, 21 YEARS OLD

Key issues: inadequate personality disorder and practical goal setting.

Summary of history

Phillip is admitted to an acute unit having attempted suicide with an aspirin overdose. He does not know why he did this, except that he felt confused and uncertain about his future, having just completed his university degree. On more detailed assessment it is found that he has a distant relationship with his parents who lead active business–social lives, but a close relationship with their live-in housekeeper. Having spent his first year of university in a hall of residence, Phillip had moved back to live at home, where his food/laundry needs were supplied.

Team strategy

The psychiatrist sees Phillip for individual psychotherapy and also sees him with the social worker for a few family therapy meetings. It is decided that the occupational therapist should help Phillip with his practical coping skills.

Initial occupational therapy assessment

Phillip presents as being passive, lacking initiative and dependent on others. On interview he says he 'should be man enough' to live independently, but feels unable to do so. He does not know what he wants to do in the future, and feels he has little control over it, except that he agrees that he wants to live rather than to die. His degree was a good one, but in life he feels a failure. A practical group cooking session shows Phillip's skills to be limited to egg-on-toast, though he enjoys the experience of both working in a group and producing a lunch. An 'interest checklist' demonstrates that Phillip has a number of slight interests such as art, cooking and stamp collecting, but he has not pursued any hobby seriously.

Treatment planning

What	How
1. Encourage sense of agency and personal responsibility	Regular setting of his own goals with practical emphasis
2. Increase practical and domestic independence skills	(a) Regular cooking group sessions to learn and practise skills; (b) attendance once-weekly at 'life skills' group — encompassing discussion, support and practical tasks
3. Raise confidence in self as an effective, competent and independent person	
4. Encourage realistic planning for the future — regarding jobs, living independently, developing outside social contacts, etc.	Once-weekly one-to-one behavioural counselling to set goals and consider life options

Progress of treatment

The key to Phillip's long-term treatment was the practical goal setting which he negotiated weekly with the occupational therapist. He found that having a goal in written form helped to make it a concrete realistic possibility, and also having to 'feedback' the results, ensured he fulfilled the goal. Some examples of goals he attempted latterly included:

1. Visit one specific art exhibition of choice;
2. Investigate possible day/night classes on offer in the area;
3. Sign up with the local cookery course and make arrangements for attendance;
4. Cook a complete meal for the family;
5. Investigate possible places to live for the future, comparing options, prices and viability, prior to discussion in the 'life skills' group.

Phillip was discharged as an in-patient after a fortnight, but continued to attend sessions as a day-patient. He eventually found his own place to live (whilst maintaining social contacts with his family), and was beginning to look for a job when he was discharged.

Discussion

The use of goal-setting in Phillip's treatment is primarily a behavioural strategy, but also has its roots in a humanistic approach. Specific behavioural targets are systematically drawn up to act as a motivator, providing both an end goal towards which to strive, and a reinforcement when achieved. The technique is an effective one to modify behaviour, providing realistic and measurable goals are attempted. Most important, however, the patient needs to be involved in their design, and be the one to identify when he or she is ready to move on to another goal. Herein lies the humanistic shadings, with Phillip being active in his own treatment, and also respected as the best judge of what is needed and when.

CASE STUDY 6 — FRAN, 15 YEARS OLD

Key issues: behaviour and family problems, creative therapy.

Summary of history

Fran is admitted to an adolescent unit as a day patient, with a history of behaviour problems and suspected substance abuse. Her parents report that she is out of their control with her rebellious, abusive behaviour. On occasions, for example, she has stayed out all night, coming home drunk. Fran's frequent arguments with her parents usually culminate in her locking herself in her room for hours, saying her parents do not understand her. At school her behaviour also seems problematic, as she is described as 'part of the deviant group who play truant and take drugs'.

Team strategy

The unit, running on therapeutic community lines, works with Fran primarily in groups, and with her family. Aside from the general ward community meetings where often the adolescents 'control' each other, a number of set groups are held daily, which the residents are expected to attend. The three main types of groups offered are:

1. Psychotherapy groups (projective art, dramatherapy or small group discussions);
2. Life skills groups (social skills training and educational groups);
3. Work groups (woodwork, cooking or sports).

The doctors and social worker are involved in family therapy. The doctors, psychologist and occupational therapist lead the psychotherapy groups. The nurses, teachers and occupational therapist run the more practical groups.

Initial occupational therapy assessment

The first fortnight of Fran joining the community activities is the assessment period, as opposed to formal one-to-one procedures. Specific tools used within the groups are projective art, 'draw your family', and self-identity self-rating questionnaires. Key points from the assessment findings include:

1. Feelings — Fran shows herself to be angry and frustrated with her family and situation, whilst also being unhappy and uncertain about her own identity. She feels that her parents hate her and see her as a failure. On her part, she wishes they were not so old and lacking in understanding. Fran feels worthless in herself except when 'with her friends or high on drugs'.
2. Behaviour — Fran finds authority and assertion situations particularly difficult. In both, she escalates the situation and becomes aggressive/abusive. She also seems to have limited internal controls, resulting in 'acting-out' behaviour. She gets on well with her peers, though as a leader is occasionally inclined to bully others. On the other hand she is skilled in many ways, having a sense of humour, being quick-thinking and also creative.

Treatment planning

What	How
1. Explore angry, ambivalent feelings about her parents	Once-weekly closed group of projective art
2. Raise esteem in herself as a worthy person	(a) All group work highlighting her strengths and assets; (b) success experience in daily printing and magazine class
3. Encourage her self-awareness	Once-weekly dramatherapy session using mainly interaction games and role play
4. Help her recognise the differences between aggression and assertion	

Progress of treatment

Fran's stay at the day unit was primarily an opportunity 'to grow' and 'time out' from the vicious cycle of negative experiences with which she was involved. She gained much self-awareness and a positive self-esteem from the community experiences. In projective art, for example, Fran expressed a number of aggressive, destructive feelings (e.g. 'what I am like inside' painting), but she also had the opportunity to explore what she liked about herself. This latter activity she initially found difficult to do, but gradually, after several similar activities, she was able to admit positive things about herself. In dramatherapy Fran enjoyed the close group work and fun of the lively games. She also eventually came to share much of her feelings about her family. One significant activity was her family 'sculpt', looking at her family in the present and who she would like them to be. This opened up several scenarios of how Fran could help bring the two images closer together. The regular family therapy sessions were also a significant growth point for Fran, with the opening up of generational communication and negotiating the giving of more positive things to each other. Fran attended the day hospital full-time for two months, and then one day a week for the next three months, as she returned to school. During this latter period much use was made of follow-up work, and contracts to encourage her motivation to attend school and make it a constructive experience.

Discussion

In Fran's treatment, projective art was a central activity. The occupational therapist who used this medium drew on a psychodynamic and humanistic approach. At the analytical end of the spectrum the art was used as a means of tapping unconscious material and as a way of channelling aggressions (through projection). On the humanistic side Fran was encouraged to explore her self concept (particularly the positive aspects) and exercise her creativity. In this case study the two approaches were able to coexist to an extent, but treatment stands in danger of being uncomfortably contradictory as the focus of the two approaches is different, with the analytical referring to the past and unconscious material, and humanism highlighting the spontaneous expressions of the here-and-now. Most therapists will have their own aims which implicitly selects one or other approach (e.g. projection = analytical, self-awareness = humanism).

CASE STUDY 7 — JOE, 70 YEARS OLD

Key issues: senile dementia, assessment, reality orientation.

Summary of history

Joe, a bachelor, is admitted to an assessment unit for the elderly, with a diagnosis of senile dementia. Whilst being physically healthy, he has a one year history of increasing forgetfulness and being unsafe at home. His neighbours and the social worker report that he has frequently wandered, or got lost while out shopping. The warden in his warden-controlled flat reports he is unsafe, as he left the gas on. She also says that Joe is socially isolated except for his regular contacts with his home help and meals-on-wheels.

Team strategy

The nurses and the occupational therapist are the key people involved in assessing Joe's functioning to consider whether to return him home or to apply for Part III accommodation. The ward also operates a continuous reality orientation programme and, as such, the team's approach to Joe needs to be consistent, reinforcing relevant information such as where he is, and the time of day. The nursing staff play a key role in Joe's daily management, whilst the occupational therapist runs a range of activity groups.

Initial occupational therapy assessment

Assessment was carried out using the standardised CAPE assessment (see Chapter 3) plus general observation in tasks and activity sessions on the ward. The findings can be summarised as:

1. Behaviour — Joe presents as having a well-preserved

115

personality, being friendly, with a sense of humour, and looking clean and tidy in dress. Whilst able to interact politely with others, he finds carrying out a conversation difficult (see below).

2. Cognitive — Joe is disorientated in time and place. His recent recall is impaired but he has a fair long-term memory. In tasks he gets confused using tools, and is easily distracted with poor concentration (less than five minutes). Joe exhibits some expressive and receptive language difficulties, and he finds it easier to respond to visual cues than answering direct questions.

3. Feelings — occasionally Joe will become aggressive, or indicate that he is frustrated and lacking in confidence. This occurs particularly at the times when he has insight into his problems. Mostly, however, Joe remains cheerful, and open to having some 'gentlemanly fun'.

Treatment planning

What	How
1. With a view to returning to his flat, assess safety and ability in: using the gas fire, making tea, and using the intercom (as required for his particular complex). With a view to Part III, ensure independence in mobility and self-care.	Practical assessments using appropriate tools
During hospital stay:	
2. Attempt to maintain or improve disorientation, confusion and memory loss	(a) Staff approach; (b) daily reality orientation session reinforcing main information
3. Maintain/improve task performance skills	Two daily activity sessions involving familiar crafts, card games, dominoes and light physical exercise

IMPLEMENTATION OF TREATMENT

What	How
4. Provide social involvements	Use of group/social activities, especially dance and music
5. Activate long-term memories and stimulate more recent recollections	Reminiscence therapy using photographs, music and limited discussion, ensuring present-day orientation
6. Maintain dignity and sense of individuality (giving him a role and bringing in personal belongings)	Put Joe in charge of watering plants, including two of his own special ones; staff approach also important

Progress of treatment

Within the first month of Joe's admission the team recommended him for Part III accommodation as his cognitive difficulties made him unsafe for independent living in his previous flat. Joe remained in the unit for a year, whilst his waiting list place came through. For the most part he seem to enjoy the social contact and stimulation in the unit. His final assessment prior to discharge indicated a slight improvement in his social ability, and only minimal deterioration in his cognitive functioning. He remained independent in mobility and self-care.

Discussion

In psychiatry dealing with the long-stay population, and when working with elderly people, occupational therapists often deal with continuing handicaps where the possibility of deterioration is a constant reality against which we battle. As a result of this, most of our aims revolve around maintaining function rather than improving it. For some this can seem unsatisfying, boring, or a waste of our time and resources. For others it is exciting work, made meaningful by setting realistic small objectives, and the feeling of performing a worthwhile job. The fact that existing demographic trends are leading to a vastly increased elderly population alerts us to the need to examine our attitudes to working with the longer-stay elderly.

CASE STUDY 8 — MARGE, 40 YEARS OLD

Key issues: manic depression, domestic role, time structuring.

Summary of history

Marge is referred to the local day hospital for treatment with a diagnosis of manic depression. She has recently been in a depressed phase where she simply lay in bed all day. This culminated in her taking an overdose of sleeping pills which her husband discovered. On other occasions Marge had become excessively active, doing domestic chores around the house, showing also a difficulty in pacing herself and activities, with her tendency to collapse at the end of the day. Marge was first diagnosed as having manic depression two years previously, when her only son went off to college. She became distraught at losing him, maintaining he was her reason for living. When he left, she still kept up with cleaning his room and cooking his meals daily. Marge has a strained relationship with her husband, which is made worse as a result of him being at home all day (as he was made redundant this year).

Team strategy

Marge's extreme mood swings are controlled by medication. The social worker and psychiatrist are additionally involved in doing marital therapy. The team agreed that the occupational therapist should help Marge with her role at home and daily time structuring.

Initial occupational therapy assessment

Marge is assessed over a few weeks using a range of tools, e.g. interview and observation, self-rating scales for daily timetable (past and present), hobby/interest checklist, cooking task-group, home visit. The following interlinked problems are identified:

1. Difficulty in planning realistic (and balanced) daily timetable;
2. Lack of acceptance of son not living at home with the attached implications of her lessened role;
3. Habits and mental set of working for others to the point of exhaustion, rather than giving space for herself;
4. Lack of social contacts or interests/hobbies outside of domestic role and family.

On her strength side she has shown much ability and knowledge of houseworking skills, and is basically kind and helpful to others. She also receives some emotional and social support from her family.

Treatment planning

What	How
1. Develop her ability to plan a realistic and balanced timetable (aiming to continue such a routine in the long term)	Daily timetable and weekly activities programme to be regularly negotiated
2. Raise her esteem in herself as a person	Involvement in a range of activities/groups offering success experience new relationships, e.g. relaxation and dance, and helping 'co-run' the cookery group.
3. Help her to develop a hobby interest which she can pursue in the long term	Dressmaking class (her choice)

Progress of treatment

Marge greatly enjoyed her time at the day hospital and participating in the activities. To this end she eventually joined the 'ex-patients' activities club, which met once weekly. Initially she was uncertain and lacking in confidence in learning dressmaking, but this became an exciting project, involving fabric printing, and making clothes for herself, her family and some hospital friends. She also pursued her new interest in joining a local dressmaking class which further increased her skills. However, Marge's timetabling skills remained problematic, and she continued to need prompting, to contain her activities, and help, to negotiate a balanced programme (e.g. from husband or therapist). This role was eventually taken up by her husband, who also participated in planning his daily routine. After a year of day hospital attendance Marge was discharged fully. She seemed happier and more confident with her fuller life and skills, though she remained somewhat vulnerable, with her mood swings. One important conflict worth noting, that the team faced throughout treatment, was to not overstep the boundaries of trying to change Marge's values of her domestic role, but rather to work within them.

Discussion

This case example highlights a common aspect in much of occupational therapy in psychiatry. We often deal with serious psychiatric illnesses, where the prognosis regarding relapse ranges from fair to poor. This may make us question the value of our treatment. At these times we need to return to the idea that we do not treat a diagnosis, but instead attempt to help in a range of problem areas. Hopefully, our choice of priority problems to tackle will have a relevant impact on the person's future capacities. In Marge's case the occupational therapist was not in a position to do much about the illness of manic depression. Treatment instead had a more limited aim; namely helping Marge manage her time/behaviour better, within the larger context of her role at home.

7

Evaluation

Evaluation is often considered to be the last stage of the occupational therapy process. Strictly speaking this is inaccurate, as we should be concerned throughout treatment to review our performance, in order to ensure the maintenance of good standards of occupational therapy practice. Indeed, this applies throughout our professional development and constitutes what is termed our 'quality assurance'.

What is involved in evaluation? Broadly speaking we can identify three key areas: (a) reviewing the treatment process; (b) reporting any results; (c) research — the long-term evaluation. Each of these areas has its critical role to play in our occupational therapy service and, as such, deserves some space and attention in this chapter.

REVIEWING THE TREATMENT PROCESS

Throughout the treatment process we should be continuously evaluating its progress. This mostly occurs automatically when we monitor for particular changes or milestones as part of the treatment process itself. It should also occur formally (and regularly), where we systematically review the process of treatment as a whole. Basically, having collected and analysed data, our task is to assess the results of, and modify, the programme. Two interlinking aspects of our work need to be reviewed: (a) the patients and their treatment; (b) ourselves.

The patient and treatment

The patients and their treatment need periodic reassessment to monitor progress and incorporate new information. The results may signal the need to adjust the treatment, or may just act as an encouragement for both patient and therapist when progress is apparent. Firstly, data need to be collected, mirroring the initial assessment process with preferably the same procedures being used to allow accurate comparisons. Here we will wish to ask what is the patient's current functioning and attitude to treatment? We can then analyse the data in terms of a number of questions. What progress has been made? Have the treatment goals been achieved — if not, why not? We may also reflect on the overall treatment given, e.g. whether the activities/grading used have been effective? Lastly, we may re-formulate the programme by adjusting it to the feedback received, and accommodating it, to take account of any changes within the patient, or his or her situation.

The prerequisite for an efficient and easy evaluation of treatment lies in having originally formulated good and precise goals as opposed to more general aims. To appreciate the full impact of this, compare the following ways of formulating the same aim:

1. Improve task performance;
2. Improve ability to follow instructions;
3. Improve ability to follow written instructions, independently.

Only the last aim begins to offer the opportunity to evaluate progress. It would be even more effective to formulate this as a goal objective saying:

At the end of two weeks treatment, Mr ____ should be able to follow written instructions for a basic woodwork task, independently.

This goal is fruitful on evaluation, as the criteria for successful achievement are clearly stated. The therapist and patient who had only aimed to 'improve task performance' may well be left uncertain as to whether or not any gains have been realised.

Ourselves

Sometimes we are so busy assessing and caring for patients that we forget to assess and care for ourselves. Whilst reflecting on our own abilities, attitudes and actions is an anxiety-provoking business, it is also crucial to our ability to work effectively in the long term. 'The most important prerequisite to being an effective helper is self-knowledge' (Hopkins and Tiffany, 1983: 94). In essence, we monitor ourself to ensure standards of our past actions, gain support if needed for present activity, and as a learning process for the future. In understanding self-appraisal there are some obvious questions that we need to ask. Was my assessment of the patient fairly objective, with judgements backed by evidence? Did I have a clear overall view of treatment and proceed accordingly? Are my attitudes to my patient appropriate, or are negative feelings (e.g. pessimism, even hostility) getting in the way? Have I carried out the necessary team liaison to maintain relationships? What are my special strengths that I offer as a therapist?

One vital question, which may well get forgotten, is: Am I arranging adequate support and supervision to ensure that I work competently? I think it is essential for all therapists to have some individual, or group, to whom they can turn on a regular basis. This can include one-to-one supervision sessions, team teaching seminars or 'sensitivity groups'. Sadly, many occupational therapists are working in teams that are short-staffed, and this area may not be given priority. Here the occupational therapist needs to take responsibility for her own development, and if possible arrange a supportive outlet. Given the nature of many psychiatric settings we are only able to sustain the emotional and physical assaults and demands on our psyche by attending occasionally to our own needs.

*　　*　　*

Ideally, in our treatment process, we first identify problems and then implement problem-solving strategies. In reality, treatment may not progress in the desired or anticipated manner, or new problems may emerge which require attention. The actual result is a continuous circuit in which problems, strategies and outcomes interact with each other (figure 7.1).

Figure 7.1: The problem-solving cycle

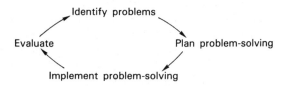

Theory into Practice
(Problem-solving and evaluation)

A case in point . . . Ben's situation is a good example of rehabilitation that lacked sufficient evaluation of a kind which might have pre-empted further 'mistakes'.

Problem situation. Ben is a 30-year-old man who has a mild mental handicap. He was brought up by his mother, living at home and attending a day centre. He functioned well and fairly independently until his mother died two years ago. Ben was taken into the local institution for shelter and with a view to rehabilitation and resettlement. After some initial 'behaviour problems', Ben settled down to the new routines of living in a supervised half-way house and working in the occupational therapy industrial therapy unit. He was well liked, and skilled and reliable in his work. After some preparation, when places came up, he was discharged to a group home in the community and a local sheltered workshop. Two weeks later Ben returned to hospital in a state of anxiety and exhibiting a range of behaviour problems.

Analysis. The treatment team carefully evaluated Ben's current situation, recognising the following problem areas:
1. Problems with Ben: anxiety; behaviour problems; sense of failure; lack of confidence; fear of the future; issues of bereavement and loss resurfaced.
2. Problems within his environment: group home residents not operating as a supportive, co-operative unit; workshop fairly pressured, with an impatient, authoritarian manager.
3. Inadequate treatment: treatment process was too quick/ not graded carefully enough with visits, overnight stays,

---

124

etc.; too many changes pushed through at once; not enough attention given to bereavement aspects of terminating hospital stay; inadequate liaison with workshop manager; inadequate follow-up support.

Problem-solving plan. In the initial stages, allow Ben the sanctuary of hospital to rebuild confidence and gain support. Gradually resettle into a group home in the middle stages, maintaining active support. He should continue working in the sheltered workshop within the hospital for security. In the late stage of rehabilitation Ben should either undergo work resettlement or return to the day centre he had attended several years previously. Careful assessment and preparation is required here.

There are a number of reasons why, on evaluation, we may find a patient has not progressed/achieved desired goals, and thus requires further intervention. Firstly, there are factors located within the individual that can influence treatment. For instance, we may encounter relapse/re-emergence of illness symptoms which interfere with functioning; or the patient may have changed/ improved markedly, rendering the treatment inappropriate; or there may be lack of motivation (as a result of illness, or attitudes in the environment). Secondly, factors concerning the patients' environment may be affecting them. Family members may be resisting treatment, contradictory staff attitudes or hostile community reactions are some key examples. Finally, the treatment team need to take some responsibility if treatment is not producing desired results. Here, we might look out for poor initial assessment, poor timing of interventions, too much stimulation/ challenge, inadequate grading, lack of team co-operation, etc.

RECORDING AND REPORTING

I earlier identified 'reporting any results' as the second key area of evaluation. Now, it may seem to you that communicating treatment is not strictly evaluation. However, I wish to argue that it is an extremely helpful tool in the process. Indeed, it is so crucial to our work that it needs special note. Recording and reporting (particularly report writing) are no-one's favourite tasks — indeed some of us may avoid doing it at all! — and yet it is a critical aspect of our job for both the present and the future. For the here-and-now, reports are essential as a means of communication with other team members. Without this we are working in a vacuum where, at best, this means we lose out on support, and at worst it could be dangerous (for the patient or ourselves), if team members are not clear about the picture. Clear communications — both written and spoken — have the additional advantage of promoting our profession, gaining us greater credibility. Professional-looking reports will bring a clearer picture of our role into the limelight by offering regular illustrations of what we actually do. Our team liaison and relationships cannot help but be improved with this sort of attention to our reports, to say nothing of the improvement for the patient's care, if we are working as an effective team. Keeping records and writing reports are also helpful for us as a 'self-disciplining' exercise, since it makes us sit down and reflect on, and evaluate, our treatments.

From a longer-term perspective there are numerous occasions when having a past treatment record is important. Take the situation of the patient who has been readmitted. Is it not dreadful to have no record at all of his or her months of intensive and perhaps successful treatment? It is not uncommon to have only the initial report, with no record of treatment, end-functioning, discharge recommendations, etc. In these situations it is the patient who suffers. Past records are also useful for the data they provide for research (e.g. follow-up studies or quality assurance projects such ˉ as recording treatment time from referral to discharge). Finally, having accurate records to refer back to, is vital, if any legal or litigation situations should arise (e.g. a patient denying he or she has had advice).

Let us look at some aspects of written and spoken reports in a little greater detail.

Written reports

In terms of evaluating a patient's treatment we write (or should!) four main types of reports:

1. Initial assessment report — this is a summary of the assessment

findings (possibly with attached assessment forms as appendices), and should include an outline plan of intervention, i.e. aims, short- and long-term goals.

2. Progress report — this should be written after each formal reassessment, or any particular alterations in treatment. It may be only a short paragraph, highlighting the relevant points.

3. Discharge summary — out of all the reports this is the most crucial one, as it states:
   a) what has happened throughout treatment,
   b) the patient's functioning and attitudes on discharge,
   c) what future occupational therapy contact should entail,
   d) any recommendations (this last point may be especially critical regarding the future health of the patient so it must be stressed in black and white).

4. Special reports — these include the specific reports that may be requested (e.g. for a special school or work unit), but also cover the little notes we must write reporting particular events or unusual happenings.

Typical areas which deserve to be recorded are: accidents or violent incidents, threats of suicide or to leave the hospital, epileptic seizures, and marked behaviour or mood swings. This is all vital information which the team must have as a written record, rather than as casual comment which can be easily forgotten. The report should be dated and should briefly describe the event/what happened and the context, and then signed.

With regard to how to write a report, all of these need to follow the same principles, namely:

1. Know the reader's needs. What information does the reader need to have? What will help the reader pick up the information easily?

2. Be clear. Use headings, lists and spacing to organise the information. Write in a succinct manner. Be legible.

3. Be thorough. Have all the main points been covered? Does the reader need any other information?

4. Date and sign the report, noting your name and position.

Report writing is a skill, and like any other form of communication it takes practice to do it well. The first initial assessment report I wrote took me 5½ hours to complete! We each find our

Figure 7.2: Sample of report preparation

Name: Martin Lawrence   Age 30
Date of assessment: April 23   Method: observation in group and tasks.

General Behaviour	Interpersonal	Task Performance	Plan
Carelessly dressed	withdrawn	No interest < Task accomplishment	½ hour daily for 2 weeks
unkempt appearance	seemed unaware of others in group	Compliant	
Clothes soiled	highly pervasive	limited energy level	relationship
Needs washing/prompting to shave.	thought needs to push to get a response	Concentration v. poor	1:1 session
Sometimes both smiling/laughing inappropriately	dependent - demanding no attention.	Careless	Basic task.
No responsibility or motivation without prompting		Needed continuous prompting to attend to details	further assessment required.
preoccupied with own thoughts	Unable to carry on conversation monosyllables	needed assistance to carry out basic task re: problem solving	
Very flat expression	slow communication	lack motivation	
Hypoactive with sudden jerky movement	Ideas/thoughts	needs prompting to re-engage	
Rapid orientation.	Speech minimal in his own world	figure ground difficulty? didn't take initiative or make independent decisions	
Apparently hearing voices	group ignore him		
Unaware of self			

Figure 7.3: Initial assessment report

Name: Martin Lawrence   *Age:* 30
Date of assessment: 23 April 1987
Methods of assessment: observation in group and tasks.

General behaviour:
Mr. Lawrence presents with an unkempt appearance given his
slightly soiled clothes. Whilst generally hypoactive, he makes
sudden jerky movements. This ties in with his occasionally bizarre
behaviour of smiling or laughing inappropriately. His non-verbal
expression tends to be flat at other times.

Interpersonal behaviour:
On observing Mr. Lawrence in a small task group, his withdrawn
highly passive behaviour is marked. He seems unaware of others
in the group (who tend to ignore him) and remains preoccupied
with his own thoughts. His communication skills are currently
poor as he has difficulty in carrying out a casual conversation, and
only expresses himself in monosyllables when pressed by the
therapist.

Task performance:
Mr. Lawrence currently shows a great deal of difficulty when
performing a basic task of either making a leather belt or baking
scones. His concentration is poor affecting overall performance.
Whilst engaged in a small 10 minute task his attention wandered
several times and he needed prompting to re-engage in the
activity. He has difficulty in following verbal instructions, and
requires repetition and demonstration. Mr. Lawrence required
assistance to problem-solve and attend to details. Overshadowing
all of these aspects is his lack of motivation to engage in the task
which required continual therapist prompting. Whilst he seems to
have no interest in his accomplishment he compliantly followed
both tasks through.

Conclusions:
On initial assessment, Mr. Lawrence has shown extreme
difficulties in all areas of functioning. Key problem areas
concerning occupational therapy are:
passive behaviour
poor social skills
poor task performance skills influenced largely by problems of
concentration and motivation.

Provisional treatment plan:
In view of the acute nature of his illness, and his current
performance difficulties, occupational therapy input will be limited
to ½ hour daily one-to-one sessions. Emphasis of treatment will
be on attempting to establish a therapeutic relationship and to
encourage Mr. Lawrence to actively engage in basic tasks. This
plan is subject to a review after further assessment in two weeks.

Signed: Karen Anders

Position: Basic grade occupational therapist

own methods. Mine, which you may find useful, is: first to devise headings; then brainstorm the possible content; after that select the good and eliminate the unnecessary points; finally formulate sentences and produce report (see figures 7.2 and 7.3). One very useful way of finding our own style is to use every opportunity to study 'good' reports by others, and to get some feedback/supervision on the ones you write.

Verbal reports

The principles of good verbal reporting follow the lines of written reporting in trying to be clear and succinct. Two other ideas which may be helpful are:

1. Be prepared — have notes written down (on e.g. patients' progress or arguments as to why they should not be discharged) prior to the meeting;
2. Listen to the reports of others to tie into, or perhaps even challenge, the information they offer.

The situations which require us to make a formal verbal report — for example ward rounds and case conferences — are often important for their information-sharing and decision-making function. It can be critical for the patient's future that we get our information right and accurate, focusing on the essentials. Finally, our own professional reputation is on the spot in a very immediate way — an additional reason to give a good account of ourselves.

RESEARCH

Finally we come to our third key area of evaluation — research. Engelhardt has asserted that 'The unexamined profession is not worth practising' (Yerxa, 1986: 209), and this is as much true of occupational therapy as any other professional group. The importance of research, as a way of examining and substantiating our practice and retaining professional credibility, cannot be overstated. Researchers contribute to our profession by developing our knowledge and guiding our theory, and in turn this helps us to refine our skills and evaluate our practice. Research also has a way of questioning and challenging current, accepted practice, which can make us feel uneasy, and yet it is also that which challenges us to improve our service. Whilst not every occupational therapist will wish to be a 'research producer', we should all have a nodding acquaintance with its methods as a 'consumer'. In this sense research is within the reach and capabilities of all occupational therapists, however inexperienced we may be. This section will examine both the consumption and production of research, and give some relevant references for those wishing to go further.

On being a research consumer

The first step on the ladder of 'doing research' is being an interested consumer. Regularly reading (and critically analysing) various research papers is an excellent way of both tuning into current issues and grappling with the methods, jargon and concepts of research. A good place to start for the uninitiated is the *British Journal of Occupational Therapy*, which regularly publishes a research paper. Also note other occupational therapy journals from for instance, the United States (e.g. the *American Journal of Occupational Therapy* and the *Occupational Therapy Journal of Research*), Canada and Australia. Other journals/periodicals (e.g. those from nursing, psychiatry and the social sciences) also offer much that is potentially exciting and relevant. Sadly, the notions of literature searches or coping with library technology can seem a daunting prospect for the uninitiated. But it gets easier as you work at it and, once mastered, the pursuit of questions and answers can be fun.

A little practical experience of academic situations, combined with some knowledge of basic methodology, is all that is necessary to be able to digest critically much of the research relevant to us. Sometimes the hardest aspect is to judge whether a particular report is a reputable one. For this, look for the following points:

1. Are the objectives clearly spelt out?
2. Do the methods used achieve them?
3. The theoretical assumptions being made; are they clearly identified and acknowledged?
4. Is the sample group suitably representative?

131

5. Are the results clearly charted?
6. Is the discussion relevant to the results?
7. Are the conclusions linked to the results?
8. Has a clear bibliography been given?
9. Is it a useful, relevant or interesting project? This last question signals the danger of researching what is measurable, rather than what is meaningful.

On being a research producer

Occupational therapy research is still in its early stages (particularly in the United Kingdom), but it is an area that is fast-expanding as more of us get involved. Increasingly, occupational therapists are gaining research experience, both in pursuit of higher degrees, and also because of the changes that have occurred in our basic training, where research is now automatically included. This is set within the backdrop of pressure to produce evidence for, and to evaluate our service in response to, quality assurance programmes.

So what research can we usefully carry out? A wide range of different types of research is possible (see figure 7.4); which method is used depends of course on the type of study. Consider the following examples for some ideas of what could be valuably used:

1. Contrast two groups of patients — one group who are engaged full-time in occupational therapy activities, the other group (control) who are on the ward full-time without structured activity. If carefully set up, e.g. balancing variables, this could be a useful demonstration of the value of occupational therapy.
2. Do a descriptive study comparing the activities available in day centres in different areas. This could be useful for providing new ideas and as a management exercise.
3. Consider a longitudinal study of what happens to patients pre- and post-discharge to the community. One possible line of enquiry would be to compare how they envisaged discharge with the actual outcome three months later.
4. Design, pilot and standardise an assessment tool for your unit's use. Much work is involved to ensure that you do it

Figure 7.4: Summary of main forms of research

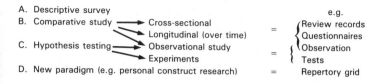

A. Descriptive survey

B. Comparative study ⟶ Cross-sectional
                   ↘ Longitudinal (over time)

C. Hypothesis testing ⟶ Observational study
                   ↗ Experiments

D. New paradigm (e.g. personal construct research)

e.g.

= { Review records / Questionnaires

= { Observation / Tests

= Repertory grid

'properly', but it provides a valuable end product.

5. Devise a questionnaire checking out attitudes/views of occupational therapy or other aspects.

These are just a few ideas — all of which are likely to be of interest and possibly of use to the rest of our profession.

How do we carry out research? The process is a complex one requiring much organisation and knowledge of correct method. Thus it is always best, for the first time at least, to be well supervised or work with an experienced colleague/team. At the end of the day you should be able to answer, coherently, the following questions:

Questions	*Sections in your report*
Why did I start?	Introduction and objectives
What did I do?	Methodology
What answer did I get?	Results and analysis
What does it mean?	Discussion and conclusions

Theory into Practice
(Summary of 'how to do research')

I Background thinking/organisation:
    — read around the subject, refine ideas;
    — decide on research question and design;
    — carry out necessary liaison.

II Prepare research method:
    — consider methods, resources, reliability, validity;
    — prepare measurement tools.

133

III Collect data:
  — run pilot and make adjustments;
  — collect real data ensuring accuracy and ethical aspects
    (e.g. confidentiality, not harming patients, their
    rights to privacy, etc.).

IV Analyse results:
  — explain clearly by using relevant tables, graphs,
    statistical analysis, etc.;
  — recognise implications.

V Present results:
  — write up in the following format: title, abstract,
    introduction and relevant literature, procedures and
    methods, results, discussion, conclusion and
    references.

For further details a useful textbook is Partridge and
Barnitt, (1986).

One last point to stress, concerning being a research producer,
is the importance of publishing any research. A researcher may
feel she or he is taking a risk of having her or his work open to
scrutiny by others — but even if the feedback is critical, will this
not be useful for future projects? Furthermore, it is only through
publishing our material that we can share our knowledge and
labours, gaining from each other. For those interested, copies of
published theses (Fellowship and MSc), written by occupational
therapists, are available from the College of Occupational
Therapists, 20 Rede Place, London, W2 4TU.

For the future

For the future we can anticipate exciting initiatives with expand-
ing research practice, from those who are enthusiastic about this
way of examining and evaluating our work. Yerxa has written
(Hopkins and Smith, 1983: 872) about the 'evolution of professional knowledge which proceeds from the intuitive practice of an
untested art to the logically rigorous practice of a science.'

Perhaps we should strive to achieve a balance between the two. Certainly we need to develop more reliable instruments and ways of testing our practice. At the same time we need to retain our humanistic values — we need to avoid reducing our patients to experimental subjects, and in the process losing sight of our holistic concerns. The challenge lies in finding methods to suit our practice, as well as adapting our practice in the light of the findings of our research.

DISCUSSION QUESTIONS

1. Why is it important to evaluate our practice?
2. What specific aspects of the treatment process should we evaluate?
3. What specific tools are available for evaluating treatment?
4. It is essential, for our future as a profession, that occupational therapists carry out research. Discuss.
5. Critically evaluate an occupational therapy report written in a patient's case notes.
6. Critically evaluate a newly published research article of interest.

8

Present and Future Trends

In recent years many forces have contributed to a reshaping of our wider health care service. Changing demographics, political debates on the economics and role of the health service, the rise of new technology and changes in education are but a few important examples. These shifts have also affected occupational therapy, where we have absorbed the changes and new developments. We have adapted both our attitudes and practice in ways that have sometimes been difficult, but also at times have put us at the front of innovation. Many of these current and future trends in both wider health care and occupational therapy have been touched on in earlier chapters. This chapter aims to highlight still further some of these aspects, in an attempt to stimulate reflection and discussion on these important issues. It is an opportunity to articulate both the problems and pressures we face, and indicate the excitements and opportunities they open up for us. By giving these points an airing we will, at the very least, be more aware of issues affecting us, and at best we may be able to deal more efficiently with any adjustments that need to be made.

In an effort to explore some current and future trends I have selected four themes for discussion: the first two relate to trends towards both a more systematic and more person-centred practice; the third raises questions concerning changes in our function and role; the fourth stresses the need to continue to promote occupational therapy to the wider world.

TOWARDS A MORE SYSTEMATIC PRACTICE?

In this era of greater accountability we are frequently being asked to justify our work and assure its quality. In practice this means that we need to be specific about our aims, carry out treatments in a coherent manner and evaluate our service in a comprehensive way. It also requires us to emphasise the value of the contributions our profession makes to health care, and to communicate this as clearly as possible when we come to present reports and argue for more resources. These are becoming imperatives, and point to the need to be more systematic in our work and more scientific in our methodology.

Said quickly, all this sounds easy. And yet buried underneath are complexities which pose many problems. Let us start with the notion of quality assurance. This phrase is being used with increasing frequency in the health service, and draws on models of efficiency, productivity and higher standards of service derived from industry. Certainly there are some parallels between industry and occupational therapy. Both need efficient organisation and require clear objectives against which to evaluate their work. Yet there are also important differences between commercial systems of production and a caring service which should not be ignored; for example the divergence in our focus on products versus patients.

A major hurdle we face, in attempting to assure quality, is to identify precisely what we are trying to do. There are two reasons why this is so difficult. Firstly, our practice is so diverse, given our varying theoretical bases, roles, concerns and work contexts. This means the answer to 'what is occupational therapy?' is highly problematic. Secondly, it is not an easy task to quantify our therapeutic input, given that we deal with many largely unquantifiable processes and lack some basic tools for accurate measurement. How can we define our approach to individual patients? How can we adequately measure the social and affective aspects of the therapy process? Can we even identify what particular aspect of our use of activity is therapeutic? These are some of the difficulties we face, particularly in psychiatry, when attempting to specify our service in 'quality assurance' terms.

However, to argue that our work cannot easily be defined, monitored or measured does not mean that we should not try to make an effort in this direction where it is appropriate to do so. There are, for example, some obvious and concrete tasks that we can undertake for ourselves as a profession, which will ultimately lead to an improvement in our service to our patients. Consider the following injunctions:

1. Be clear and systematic when we are identifying patients' problems and the aims and methods of their treatment.
2. Develop the tools to measure those aspects of our work which are open to quantification and scaling, e.g. standardised assessments are a means of enabling us to more accurately identify patients' functioning and measure improvements.
3. Record and report information more accurately and more often — taking the risk of having our work open to scrutiny by others.
4. Encourage the development of research to both substantiate our present and direct our future practices, in a more theoretically sophisticated and scientifically justifiable way.
5. At its most general, reflect on the role and practice of occupational therapy and take the opportunities to discuss and debate the state of our profession and the shape of its future development. Do you have any other ideas? If so, how will you promote them.?

TOWARDS A MORE PERSON-CENTRED PRACTICE?

If we need to move towards becoming more scientific in our approach to occupational therapy, we need simultaneously to focus on the 'person' behind the patient — paying increasing attention to his or her individuality, rights and needs.

This can be seen at several levels. Firstly we need to move away from depersonalising labels and blanket diagnoses. Instead we should pay more attention to the individual's situation and recognise that illness is only one small aspect of the whole person. When we do use a diagnosis we need to try to preserve the human element in our definitions and our verbal usages. Consider the simple but profound difference between saying 'the person with a diagnosis of schizophrenia', as against 'that schizophrenic'. Behind this difference in semantics lies some very important differences in attitudes towards concepts of health and illness, and the extent to which the physical, emotional and social impact of our treatments are taken into account.

A further key part of this recognition of the individual is our increasing awareness of the need to plan an individualised treatment, based on an assessment of a person's specific needs. The days when we received blanket referrals for all patients to attend the department, for whatever activity currently in progress, are numbered. Whilst limited resources may hamper the extent to which individual treatment planning is possible for all patients, some attempts to move in this direction must be made. Many departments, for example, now run a range of activities into which patients are carefully and selectively referred. Increasingly we are trying to fit our service to the patient, rather than patients into our service.

Another facet of this recognition of the specificity of an individual's situation is also the need to acknowledge the differences between people's social and cultural background. Many occupational therapists now work in multi-cultural areas, where it is vital they are aware of particular needs of certain groups (e.g. religious customs and taboos). Equally, we need to consider the impact of class, gender, race and age on a person's life chances, given the widespread patterns of disadvantage and even discrimination that exist with regard to them. We need to take all this into account, if we are going to plan treatments that are both relevant and realistic in today's climate.

Lastly, the patient also needs to be seen as a key member of the treatment team. Fundamental to this notion is the need to plan treatment with our patients, rather than regard them as the passive recipients of our service. This concept can be taken further to stress the importance of the idea of offering patients choices. This is a particularly acute issue when a patient is being forced against his or her will to come to occupational therapy, or is coerced into activity. This is clearly undesirable, and alerts us to the need to ask ourselves what the patient sees as 'in his or her interest', as well as reviewing what we think is in the best interests of that patient. Of course, we often have to deal with problems of lack of motivation, but there comes a point when a therapist's persuasions need to give way to the decision of the patient. Ultimately, all our patients need to have a degree of understanding of, and control over, their treatment. If our patients do not have this, they are being treated more like raw materials on a production line to be turned into an end-product of the therapist's choosing.

139

CHANGING FUNCTIONS AND ROLES?

There are many debates and concerns in our profession which continue to preoccupy us, involving questions about the direction in which occupational therapy should go in the future. And rightly so. There are two such questions which I would like to highlight here. These are — Is our profession in crisis?, and Is the nature of our practice changing?

'Is our profession in crisis?' has become a matter for vigorous debate over the past few years, particularly in the United States. Kielhofner (1983: 3–46), a key exponent of this view, argues that the crisis arises from our confused and diverse practice. This has resulted in a loss of identity for occupational therapy and its fragmentation into too many competing schools of practice. He proposes that our crisis can only be resolved by a scientific revolution where occupational therapists re-organise their professional knowledge and practice around a unified set of beliefs — for instance, that occupation is a central determinant of health. Such a debate confronts us with the need to actively consider whether we view a 'one-theory' profession as desirable or possible. Can we find a guiding framework which attracts us all? Or do we want to maintain a plurality of theoretical frameworks to reflect our diverse practice? In this situation, can we embrace a unified occupational therapy framework whilst retaining our other theories for the treatment methods they offer?

A similar debate is occurring over the use of generalist (Jack-of-all-trades) versus specialist occupational therapists. On one hand the conception of a generalist therapist is true to many of our basic values, but on the other hand it may stand in danger of offering a service that is too vague. In contrast to this, specialists may have their deeper knowledge and skills, but their move away from the basics of occupational therapy may result in a further fragmentation of our profession. Is the benefit worth the cost?

These issues will continue to be explored and argued about, and no easy answers are currently available. My own view is that we should work towards a greater unity at a grassroots level where there seems to be some consensus and mutual understanding about occupational therapy. However, if we are to develop and grow as a profession, and work co-operatively with other disciplines, we also need to develop our specialist knowledge, skills and methods. What is your view?

The second question posed above concerns the changing nature of occupational therapy practice. On the one hand most of our central values, concerns and interests, etc., reveal a considerable continuity in the history of occupational therapy. Yet there are important changes which are occurring which also need to be acknowledged. The following examples immediately come to mind:

1. There is a clearly discernible shift occurring in the forms of our applied treatment, away from work activities towards leisure concerns. Given the significant unemployment problem for the psychiatric population, many of the work therapy units have necessarily been obliged to reorganise themselves to enable patients to look at how to manage their leisure time.

2. Some moves can be detected in the direction of our vision of occupational therapy as a problem-solving process rather than a strict activity base. For example, the use of counselling techniques, giving advice, one-to-one contact in clients' homes, etc. are all more in tune with the problem-solving approach than activity-based conceptions.

3. Given the trend away from institution-based treatments towards a 'back into the community' approach, we have a new role which has not as yet been clearly defined. But such a shift may point to an increasing emphasis on helping mobilise more community and self-help supports, rather than bringing clients into hospital with all the dependence-fostering relationships this may entail.

4. Lastly, our therapeutic use of technology is increasing yearly, and this may well open up a serious and widening gap between those therapists with some technical experience and others who lack it. The currently fashionable pieces of equipment include video (e.g. in social skills training) and computers (e.g. for developing cognitive, perceptual and task skills). This, like many of the other issues raised above, has major implications for a more prominent attendance on professional updating and post-registration courses. These are some changing aspects — can you think of other shifts relevant to you?

PROMOTING OCCUPATIONAL THERAPY

There is nothing new in the felt needs to promote occupational therapy. In the past occupational therapists have been obliged to fight many battles for recognition and resources. Yet today, particularly in the context of increasing competition for limited health resources and the trend towards multi-disciplinary role-blurring, there are perhaps as great threats to our growth as a profession as have ever existed in the past. Our motive for promoting occupational therapy cannot simply be anchored in professional self-interest or our corporate history. Ultimately it is dependent upon us being proud of what we do, and wanting to share it with others.

How often do we complain about not being taken seriously as professionals? How often do we feel discouraged because occupational therapy seems undervalued, and no-one appears interested in what we say in ward rounds? Whilst the way our profession is perceived varies enormously from place to place, many of us are still in the business of challenging the false or even negative images of occupational therapy which others sometimes have. At the same time it has to be recognised that some, at least, of these negative images may be the result of the way we have presented in the past. Herein lies the need for us to promote occupational therapy — and promote it in several directions, not only towards the general public, but also and more specifically in the direction of our patients and the treatment team.

In the first instance we need to promote occupational therapy to our patients to enable them to feel reassured and clear about what they are becoming involved with. Many patients come to us with expectations that reflect the general public's limited and confused view of what we do. They may feel unsure of what it is all about, or they may be unmotivated because of some inadequate image that, for instance, 'occupational therapy is just basket-weaving'. Succinct and relevant explanations, of what occupational therapy in your unit does, should if possible be given to every patient in the early stages of treatment. A simple statement on the following lines might help both to ease any doubts the patient has about occupational therapy and perhaps actively engage their motivation and enthusiasm: 'occupational therapy is a treatment using activities. We aim to help people cope with different problems they may be having. We do lots of different things. Why not come down to the department with me and have

a look around and talk to some of the patients there?'
The rest of the treatment team also needs to know about, and
recognise the value of, occupational therapy. At one level they
are important ambassadors for us; for instance when explaining
our role to an uncertain patient. At another level the team needs
to be clear about our functions (and we about their functions) to
enable smooth liaison and co-operative effort. This task of
educating colleagues needs to be done continuously at both formal
(e.g. when presenting a report at a case conference) and informal
(e.g. when chatting casually on the ward with nurses) levels. It
is important to remember also the outward impression we may
give when we invite visitors/team members/students around the
department — additional explanations, of the aims of activities
going on, for example, are essential.

At a more instrumental or political level our image and
perceived role within a unit or hospital (and within the management hierarchy) matters if we are to maintain, or attract more of,
the resources which are necessary to enable us to do our job
effectively. Here, again, we need to communicate with others
both widely and well. Writing reports, making presentations,
holding open days, producing leaflets, etc., all involve some
degree of presenting and promoting occupational therapy to a
wider audience. And most of all, we promote our profession by
doing a good job.

*   *   *

In this and the preceding chapters we have tried to unravel some
of the complexities of our occupational therapy process, and give
examples of our work in practice. We have stressed themes such
as the need to be both systematic and scientific while also remaining person-centred and sensitive to the needs of our patients
within the treatment process. We have explored a number of the
dilemmas arising from our multi-faceted role and our wide
theoretical base. The intention has been to be informative and to
spark off some interest and debate. Throughout all of these
discussions, what has been offered is only one way of carrying
out occupational therapy in psychiatry (the way that makes sense
to me given my experiences). It does not claim to be the only
way. You may well find other, even better, ways. We are not
dealing with a clear-cut subject which has any easy or stereotyped
answers. Instead, we may take many perspectives and focus in on

143

problems and treatments at different levels.

Yes, occupational therapy in psychiatry can be utterly confusing, filled with ambiguities, contradictions, frustrations and stresses. We have relatively few answers and are often baffled by the complexities of the people and problems with which we have to deal. On the other hand, occupational therapy in psychiatry can be endlessly interesting and thought-provoking, and even fun. We can experience the sense of satisfaction and professional fulfilment when a person's treatment actually works out as we had hoped. Or sometimes the experience of a certain activity, or a relationship, feels just 'right'. We have a continuous challenge on our hands, and also rich rewards.

Appendices

APPENDIX 1: SOCIAL AND GROUP SKILLS ASSESSMENT

Name:

Date:

Other relevant information:

Observations made: over _____ (period of time)

within _____ (context/activity)

Skill area	Please place a tick in the appropriate column				
	Not observed	No problem/ appropriate	Mild problem	Severe problem, e.g. bizarre/ lack of skill	Comments
Social skills					
Conversation ability					
Non-verbal behaviour					
Sociability					
Expression of ideas, thoughts					
Group skills					
Awareness of others' needs					
Sharing behaviour					
Co-operativeness					
Independence					
Assertion/ compliance					
Competitiveness					
Role-taking ability					
Reaction to peers					
Reaction to authority					
Response to group situations					

Future plans: Signed
Position

APPENDIX 2: DOMESTIC SKILLS ASSESSMENT

Name: Address:

Date:

Home situation or domestic role:

Attitudes to domestic role:

Please rate the following skill areas as follows:-

0 = no difficulty/independent; 1 = some difficulty; 2 = considerable difficulty/unsafe. Rating should be made with reference to patient's usual routines and domestic/community facilities.

Skill areas	Patient rating	Therapist rating	Comments

1. Cooking:
    tea/coffee
    snacks
    main meals
    appropriate storage of food
    appropriate use of equipment			

2. Shopping:
    single shops
    supermarket			

3. Household chores:
    washing up
    dusting/vacuuming
    cleaning
    laundry washing
    laundry ironing
    bed making
    sewing			

4. DIY:
    fixing plugs
    handling emergencies
    house maintenance
    telephoning for services			

5. Gardening			
6. Transport/travel and community orientation			

7. Money:
    budgeting
    paying bills
    other money transactions			

Skill area	Patient rating	Therapist rating	Comments
8. Child care: feeding, dressing, toileting managing behaviour play/stimulation			
9. Family relationships: meeting others' needs meeting own needs			

Short-term treatment goals and method:

Long-term aim: Signature
                      Position
                      Date

APPENDIX 3: WORK SKILLS ASSESSMENT

Name:

Date

Work situation/Expected role:

Attitudes to work:

Please rate the following skill areas as follows:-

0 = no difficulty; 1 = some difficulty; 2 = considerable difficulty.
Comments should provide examples of, or explanations for, behaviour
noted.

Skill areas	Patient rating	Therapist rating	Comments

Task performance:
  concentration
  following instructions
    demonstrated
    verbal
    written
  speed of work
  organisation
  neatness
  accuracy
  perseverance
  problem-solving
  decision making			

Work role:
  attendance
  time-keeping
  taking responsibility
  reliability
  response to authority
  response to evaluation
  co-operation with work-mates			

Work tasks used in assessment:

Particular work skills/strength areas:

Short-term treatment goals and methods:

Long-term recommendation:

Signature

Position

Date

148

APPENDIX 4: SOCIAL SKILLS QUESTIONNAIRE*

Name: Date

Please reach each of the following statements. Rate how you handle each of these situations using the scale below:

1 = I have *no difficulty* doing this
2 = I have a *slight difficulty* doing this
3 = I have *quite a bit of difficulty* doing this
4 = I have *great difficulty* doing this
5 = I *never* do this or would *avoid* the situation

Circle the number which most closely reflects your reaction

Talking to people

1. When I meet people I can start a conversation with them
1 2 3 4 5
2. I can start talking about something and carry on a conversation
1 2 3 4 5
3. When others are talking I can join in
1 2 3 4 5
4. When someone is talking to me I can appear interested
1 2 3 4 5

Saying how I feel

1. When a person has done well I can compliment them
1 2 3 4 5
2. If someone does something for me I can thank them
1 2 3 4 5
3. I am able to encourage others
1 2 3 4 5
4. If I care about someone I can show them how I feel
1 2 3 4 5
5. I can tell someone that I am angry without losing control
1 2 3 4 5

Expressing my needs

1. I can put my point of view in an argument without losing control
1 2 3 4 5
2. I can give people instructions without feeling embarrassed
1 2 3 4 5
3. I can ask to see the person in charge if I am making a complaint
1 2 3 4 5
4. I can tell people exactly what I want (e.g. in shops)
1 2 3 4 5

Dealing with others

1. I am able to understand how other people are feeling
1 2 3 4 5
2. I can listen to what a person has to say
1 2 3 4 5
3. If I fall out with someone I can work out what went wrong
1 2 3 4 5
4. I can deal with someone who is angry without becoming upset
1 2 3 4 5

Friendship
1. I can talk to people I have met for the first time   1 2 3 4 5
2. I can talk to people in a group   1 2 3 4 5
3. I can make dates to see people   1 2 3 4 5
4. I can take the initiative to make a friendship   1 2 3 4 5
5. I can go to a new place in order to meet new people   1 2 3 4 5

Dealing with myself
1. If I am upset I can calm myself down   1 2 3 4 5
2. I can control my temper before it gets out of hand   1 2 3 4 5
3. I can make plans and stick to them   1 2 3 4 5
4. I can negotiate with people   1 2 3 4 5
5. I can work out how I feel and how I should deal with it.   1 2 3 4 5

Goals
Read over the scale again and pick out the situations which you would like to be able to deal with better. Make a list of these below.

1.

2.

3.

4.

5.

6.

___

* Assessment originally published in Barker, 1985: 236–7. Permission to reprint the form was kindly granted by Philip Barker.

Further Reading

GENERAL OCCUPATIONAL THERAPY TEXTBOOKS

Denton, P. (1987) *Psychiatric occupational therapy: a workbook of practical skills.* Little Brown, Boston.
Hopkins, H. L. and Smith, H. D. (1983) *Willard and Spackman's occupational therapy,* 6th edn. J. B. Lippincott, Philadelphia.
Kielhofner, G. (ed.) (1985) *A model of human occupation — theory and application.* Williams and Wilkins, Baltimore.
Mosey, A. C. (1986) *Psychosocial components of occupational therapy.* Raven Press, New York.
Reed, K. and Sanderson, S. (1980) *Concepts of occupational therapy.* Williams and Wilkins, Baltimore.
Willson, M. (1987) *Occupational therapy in long-term psychiatry,* 2nd edn. Churchill Livingstone, Edinburgh.

(All these texts offer a good account of both theoretical frameworks and the occupational therapy process.)

THEORETICAL FRAMEWORKS

Briggs, A. K., Duncombe, L. W., Howe, M. C. and Schwartzberg, S. L. (1979) *Case simulations in psychosocial occupational therapy.* F. A. Davis, Philadelphia.

ASSESSMENT

Barker, P. J. (1985) *Patient assessment in psychiatric nursing.* Croom Helm, London.
Hemphill, B. J. (ed.) (1982) *The evaluation process in psychiatric occupational therapy.* Charles B. Slack, New Jersey.

TREATMENT

Briggs, A. K. and Agrin, A. R. (1981) *Crossroads: a reader for psychosocial occupational therapy.* American Occupational Therapy Association, Maryland.

References

Argyle, M. (ed.) (1981) *Social skills and health*. Methuen, London.

Axline, V. (1971) *Dibs: in search of self*. Penguin, Harmondsworth.

Ayres, A. J. (1963) The development of perceptual motor abilities: a theoretical basis for treatment of dysfunction, *American Journal of Occupational Therapy*, 17, 221–5.

Baker, R. (1986) The development of a behavioural assessment system for psychiatric in-patients. Research report to the Grampian Health Board.

Barker, P. J. (1985) *Patient assessment in psychiatric nursing*. Croom Helm, London.

Briggs, A. K., Duncombe, L. W., Howe, M. C. and Schwartzberg, S. L. (1979) *Case simulations in psychosocial occupational therapy*. F. A. Davis, Philadelphia.

Coleman, P. (1986) *Ageing and reminiscence process*. John Wiley and Sons, Chichester.

Ellis, R. and Whittington, D. (1981) *A guide to social skill training*. Croom Helm, London.

Fidler, G. (1985) In Kielhofner, G. (ed.), *A model of human occupation — theory and application*. Williams and Wilkins, Baltimore.

Hemphill, B. J. (ed.) (1982) *The evaluation process in psychiatric occupational therapy*. Charles B. Slack, New Jersey.

Holden, U. and Woods, R. T. (1988) *Reality orientation*, 2nd edn. Churchill Livingstone, Edinburgh.

Hopkins, H. (1983) An historical perspective on occupational therapy. In Hopkins, H. L. and Smith, H. D. (eds), *Willard and Spackman's occupational therapy*, 6th edn. J. B. Lippincott, Philadelphia.

Hopkins, H. L. and Smith, H. D. (eds) (1983) *Willard and Spackman's occupational therapy*, 6th edn. J. B. Lippincott, Philadelphia.

Hopkins, H. L. and Tiffany, E. G. (1983) Occupational therapy – a problem-solving process. In Hopkins, H. L. and Smith, H. D. (eds), *Willard and Spackman's occupational therapy*, 6th edn. J. B. Lippincott, Philadelphia.

Jennings, S. (ed.) (1987) *Dramatherapy: theory and practice for teachers and clinicians*, Croom Helm, London.

Kielhofner, G. (ed.) (1983) *Health through occupation — theory and practice in occupational therapy*. F. A. Davis, Philadelphia.

Llorens, L. (1970) Facilitating growth and development: the promise of occupational therapy, *American Journal of Occupational Therapy*, 24, 93–101.

Mailloux, Z., Mack, W. and Cooper, C. (1983) Knowing what to do: the organization of knowledge for clinical practice. In Kielhofner, G. (ed.), *Health through occupation — theory and practice in occupational therapy*. F. A. Davis, Philadelphia.

Maslow, A. H. (1954) *Motivation and personality*. Harper and Row, New York.

152

Matsutsuyu, J. (1969) The interest checklist, *American Journal of Occupational Therapy*, 23, 323–8.

Mosey, A. C. (1986) *Psychosocial components of occupational therapy*. Raven Press, New York.

Pattie, A. H. and Gilleard, C. J. (1979) *Clifton assessment procedures for the elderly (CAPE)*. Hodder and Stoughton, London.

Partridge, C. and Barnitt, R. (1986) *Research guidelines: a handbook for therapists*. Heinemann, London.

Sieg, K. (1974) Applying the behavioural model to the occupational therapy model, *American Journal of Occupational Therapy*, 28, 421–8.

Whiting, S., Lincoln, N. B., Bhavnani, G. and Cockburn, J. (1984) *The Rivermead perceptual assessment battery*. NFER–Nelson, Windsor.

Yerxa, E. J. (1967) Eleanor Clarke Slagle Lecture: authentic occupational therapy, *American Journal of Occupational Therapy*, 21, 1–9.

—— (1983) Audacious values: the energy source for occupational therapy practice. In Kielhofner, G. (ed.) *Health through occupation — theory and practice in occupational therapy*. F. A. Davis, Philadelphia.

—— (1987) Quotations taken from talks given by Professor E. Yerxa at a conference in Exeter on 'Occupational therapy: a foundation for practice', 2–4 April.

Bibliography

Allen, C. K. (1985) *Occupational therapy for psychiatric diseases: measurement and management of cognitive disabilities.* Little, Brown, Boston.

Andrews, K. (1979) Research and the therapist, *British Journal of Occupational Therapy*, 42(2), 44–5.

Anthony, W. (1980) *The principles of psychiatric rehabilitation.* University Park Press, Baltimore.

Barris, R. (1984) Towards an image of one's own. Sources of variation in the role of occupational therapists in psycho-social practice, *Occupational Therapy Journal of Research*, 4, 3–23.

——— Kielhofner, G. and Watts, J. H. (1983) *Psychological occupational therapy: practice in a pluralistic arena.* RAMSCO, Maryland.

Bayliss, D. E., Goble, R. E. A., King, D. J. and Mendez, M. A. (1983) Present trends in occupational therapy practice, *British Journal of Occupational Therapy*, 46(8), 216–19.

Berry, R. (1978) *How to write a research paper.* Pergamon Press, Oxford.

Bolles, R. C. (1975) *Learning theory.* Holt, Rinehart and Winston, New York.

Brayman, S. J., Kirby, T. F., Misenheimer, A. M. and Short, M. J. (1976) Comprehensive occupational therapy evaluation scale, *American Journal of Occupational Therapy*, 30, 94–100.

Brechin, A. and Liddiard, P. (1981) *Look at it this way: new perspectives in rehabilitation*, Hodder and Stoughton, Sevenoaks.

Briggs, A. K. and Agrin, A. R. (1981) *Crossroads: reader for psychosocial occupational therapy.* American Occupational Therapy Association, Maryland.

Clark, P. N. (1979) Human development through occupation: theoretical frameworks in contemporary occupational therapy practice, Part 1, *American Journal of Occupational Therapy*, 33, 505–14.

——— (1979) Human development through occupation: a philosophy and conceptual model for practice, Part 2, *American Journal of Occupational Therapy*, 33, 577–85.

Cynkin, S. (1979) *Occupational therapy: toward health through activity.* Little, Brown, Boston.

Denham, M. J. (ed.) (1983) *Care of the long-stay elderly patient.* Croom Helm, London.

Denton, P. (1987) *Psychiatric occupational therapy: a workbook of practical skills.* Little, Brown, Boston.

Dexter, G. and Wash, M. (1986) *Psychiatric nursing skills: a patient-centred approach.* Croom Helm, London.

Fidler, G. S. (1981) From crafts to competence, *American Journal of Occupational Therapy*, 35, 567–73.

——— and Fidler, J. W. (1963) *Occupational therapy: a communication process in psychiatry.* Macmillan, New York.

—— and —— (1983) Doing and becoming: the occupational therapy experience. In Kielhofner, G. (ed.), *Health through occupation — theory and practice in occupational therapy*. F. A. Davis, Philadelphia.

Fransella, F. (1982) *Psychology for occupational therapists*. Macmillan, London.

Gibson, D. and Kaplan, K. (1984) *Short-term treatment in mental health*. Haworth Press, New York.

Howell, C. (1986) A controlled trial of goal setting for long-term community psychiatric patients, *British Journal of Occupational Therapy*, 49(8), 264–8.

Hughes, P. L. and Mullins, L. (1981) *Acute psychiatric care — an occupational therapy guide to exercises in daily living skills*. Slack, New Jersey.

Hume, C. and Pullen, I. (1986) *Rehabilitation in psychiatry: an introductory handbook*. Churchill Livingstone, Edinburgh.

Jennings, S. (1986) *Creative drama in groupwork*. Winslow Press, London.

Kielhofner, G. (1980) A model of human occupation, Part 2: Ontogenesis from the perspective of temporal adaptation, *American Journal of Occupational Therapy*, 34, 657–63.

—— (1980) A model of human occupation, Part 3: Benign and vicious cycles, *American Journal of Occupational Therapy*, 34, 731–7.

—— (ed.) (1985) *A model of human occupation — theory and application*. Williams and Wilkins, Baltimore.

—— and Burke, J. P. (1980) A model of human occupation, Part 1: Structure and content, *American Journal of Occupational Therapy*, 34, 572–81.

——, —— and Igi, C. H. (1980) A model of human occupation, Part 4: Assessment and intervention, *American Journal of Occupational Therapy*, 34, 777–88.

King, L. J. (1974) A sensory integrative approach to schizophrenia, *American Journal of Occupational Therapy*, 28, 529–36.

—— (1978) Towards a science of adaptive responses, *American Journal of Occupational Therapy*, 32, 429–37.

—— (1980) Creative caring, *American Journal of Occupational Therapy*, 34, 522–8.

Llorens, L. 61976) *Application of a developmental theory for health and rehabilitation*. American Occupational Therapy Association, Maryland.

Mosey, A. C. (1970) *Three frames of reference for mental health*. Charles B. Slack, New Jersey.

—— (1973) *Activities therapy*. Raven Press, New York.

—— (1985) Eleanor Clarke Slagle Lecture: A monistic or pluralistic approach to professional identity? *American Journal of Occupational Therapy*, 39, 504–9.

Neff, W. S. (1985) *Work and human behaviour*, 3rd edn. Aldine, New York.

Priestley, P. and McGuire, J. (1983) *Learning to help*. Tavistock, London.

155

Purtilo, R. (1978) *Health professional/patient interaction.* 2nd edn. W. B. Saunders, Philadelphia.

Reed, K. and Sanderson, S. (1980) *Concepts of occupational therapy.* Williams and Wilkins, Baltimore.

Reilly, M. (1962) Occupational therapy can be one of the greatest ideas of 20th century medicine, *American Journal of Occupational Therapy,* 16, 1–9.

—— (ed.) (1974) *Play as exploratory learning.* Sage Publications, Beverly Hills.

Rogers, J. C. (1982) Order and disorder in medicine and occupational therapy, *American Journal of Occupational Therapy,* 36, 29–35.

—— (1983) Eleanor Clarke Slagle Lecture — Clinical reasoning: the ethics, science, and art, *American Journal of Occupational Therapy,* 37, 601–6.

Rowan, J. (1983) *The reality game. A guide to humanistic counselling and therapy.* Routledge and Kegan Paul, London.

Simon, G. B. (ed.) (1980) *Modern management of mental handicap — a manual of practice.* MTP Press, Lancaster.

Smith, M.E. (1979) Becoming involved in research, *British Journal of Occupational Therapy,* 42, 65–6.

Target 2000: *Promoting excellence in education* (1986). American Occupational Therapy Association, Maryland.

Trower, P., Bryand, B. and Argyle, M. (1978) *Social skills and mental health.* Methuen, London.

Wallace, C. J. (1986) Functional assessment in rehabilitation, *Schizophrenia Bulletin,* 12(4), 604–30.

Willson, M. (ed.) (1984) *Occupational therapy in short-term psychiatry,* Churchill Livingstone, Edinburgh.

—— (1987) *Occuptional therapy in long-term psychiatry,* 2nd edn. Churchill Livingstone, Edinburgh.

Wing, J. K. and Brown, G. W. (1971) *Institutionalism and schizophrenia.* Cambridge University Press, Cambridge.

—— and Morris, B. (eds) (1981) *Handbook of psychiatric rehabilitation practice.* Oxford University Press, Oxford.

Yerxa, E. J. (1979) *The philosophical base of occupational therapy, in 2001 AD.* American Occupational Therapy Association, Rockville, Maryland.

—— (1983) The occupational therapist as a researcher. In Hopkins, H. L. and Smith, H. D. (eds), *Willard and Spackman's occupational therapy,* 6th edn. J. B. Lippincott, Philadelphia.

—— (1986) In *Target 2000; promoting excellence in education.* American Occupational Therapy Association, Rockville, Maryland.

Yule, W. and Carr, J. (eds) (1987) *Behaviour modification for people with mental handicaps,* 2nd edn. Croom Helm, London.

Theory into Practice Index

Index

Communication *see*
  Communication activities;
  Fidlers' psychodynamic
  approach; Reports; Social
  skills training
Communication activities 85–7
Community
  occupational therapy role 8–9,
    10, 106, 141
  resources 9
Concentration
  assessment 35–6
Conceptual model 14
Contract 108
Contraindications 82, 84, 86, 87
Cookery 81, 110–11
Coping skills 109–11
  see also Anxiety management;
    Life skills group; Social
    skills training
COTE 19, 42–3
Counselling 57, 95, 110
Crafts 83, 119–20
Creative therapy 20, 112–14
  see also Creative writing;
    Dramatherapy; Projective
    art
Creative writing 52
Crisis in profession 140
Cultural aspects 56, 139

Dance
  evaluation 84
Day hospital 100–103
Delusions
  managing behaviour 70
Dependence 7, 25, 45, 110
Developmental approach
  application 22–4
  basic concepts 21–2
  case study 27–8
  see also Group interaction
    skill; Mosey
Diagnosis 4, 138
Discussion groups 85
Disorientation
  managing behaviour 71
Domestic skills assessment
  104–5, 146–8

Domiciliary role *see* Community
Dramatherapy 85, 113–14
  see also Psychodrama; Trust
    exercises
Dyadic interaction skill 22
Dynamic unconscious 16

Ecclectic approach 30, 100
Elderly people
  occupational therapy role
    10–11, 117–18
Emotional safety 39–40, 86, 87
Environment
  therapeutic use 24, 72–3
Erikson 16
Evaluation 121–35
  evaluating treatment 122–5
Extinction 18

Family work 8, 10, 104–6, 114
Feelings
  problems of 4
Fidlers' psychodynamic approach
  16
  see also Analytical approach
Frame of reference 14
Freud 16

Gardening 81
Geriatric *see* Elderly people
Goals 65–6, 122
Goal-setting with patients 102,
  111
Grading 75, 90–94
Group interaction skill 22–4,
  74–5, 93–4
  see also Mosey
Groupwork *see* Creative therapy;
  Discussion groups; Group
  interaction skill

Hobbies *see* Interest checklist;
  Social activities
Holistic approach 2–3
Home visits 10, 104, 119
Humanistic approach
  application 20–21
  basic concepts 20
  case study 27

Validity 44, 46
Volleyball 24

Woodwork 91–2
Work *see* Industrial therapy;
  Rehabilitation; Task

performance skills; Work
  skills assessment
Work skills assessment 149

Yerxa 2, 20, 135
  see also Humanistic values